Secrets of
Success

Getting into
ACADEMIC
MEDICINE

Philip J Smith BMEDSCI (HONS) BMBS (HONS) MSc (NUTRITION) MRCP

Jasdeep K Gill MB CHB (HONS) DRCOG DFSRH DCH

Sukhjinder S Nijjer BSc (HONS) MB CHB (HONS) MRCP

Jeremy B Levy MA FHEA PHD FRCP

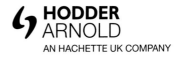

**HODDER
ARNOLD**
AN HACHETTE UK COMPANY

First published in Great Britain in 2011 by
Hodder Arnold, an imprint of Hodder Education, Hodder and Stoughton Ltd, a division of Hachette UK
338 Euston Road, London NW1 3BH

http://www.hodderarnold.com

Hachette UK's policy is to use papers that are natural, renewable and recyclable products and made from wood grown in sustainable forests. The logging and manufacturing processes are expected to conform to the environmental regulations of the country of origin.

Whilst the advice and information in this book are believed to be true and accurate at the date of going to press, neither the author[s] nor the publisher can accept any legal responsibility or liability for any errors or omissions that may be made. In particular, (but without limiting the generality of the preceding disclaimer) every effort has been made to check drug dosages; however it is still possible that errors have been missed. Furthermore, dosage schedules are constantly being revised and new side-effects recognized. For these reasons the reader is strongly urged to consult the drug companies' printed instructions before administering any of the drugs recommended in this book.

British Library Cataloguing in Publication Data
A catalogue record for this book is available from the British Library

Library of Congress Cataloging-in-Publication Data
A catalog record for this book is available from the Library of Congress

ISBN   978-1-853-15957-2

1 2 3 4 5 6 7 8 9 10

Publisher: Caroline Makepeace
Production Controller: Kate Harris
Cover Design: Lynda King
Project Managed by Naughton Project Management

Cover image © Pete Saloutos/CORBIS

The logo of the Royal Society of Medicine is a registered trade mark, which it has licensed to Hodder Arnold.

Typeset in 11/13 Minion Pro by MPS Limited, a Macmillan Company.
Printed and bound in Great Britain by CPI Antony Rowe Ltd

What do you think about this book? Or any other Hodder Arnold title?
Please visit our website: www.hodderarnold.com

To Matthew and Sarah – I love you – I told you I would mention you in the book! Beverley, Mum, Dad and all my family – thank you as always, for all your love and support in everything I do.
   PJS

To all my family, for your never-ending love and support.
   SSN

To everyone who has supported and encouraged this book.
   JKG

Karen, your books are even more exciting! (Dear reader, go and buy *The Letter in the Bottle* or *Fallen Order* by Karen Liebreich to broaden your horizons!)
   JBL

Contents

Contributors

Dr Philip J Smith BMedSci (Hons) BMBS (Hons) MSc (Nutrition) MRCP
ST4 Academic Clinical Fellow in Gastroenterology, PhD student, Medical
Research Council Clinical Research Training Fellow, University College
London, UK

Dr Jasdeep K Gill MB ChB (Hons) DRCOG DFSRH DCH
General Practice Registrar, North West Thames, London Deanery, UK

Dr Sukhjinder S Nijjer BSc (Hons) MB ChB (Hons) MRCP
Academic Clinical Fellow and Specialty Registrar in Cardiology, Imperial
College Healthcare NHS Trust and Imperial College London, UK

Dr Jeremy B Levy MA FHEA PhD FRCP
Head of the London School of Medicine and Medical Specialties, London Deanery;
Consultant Nephrologist and Physician, Imperial College Healthcare NHS Trust;
Reader in Renal Medicine and Medical Education, Imperial College London, UK

Dr Beverley Almeida BMedSci (Hons) BMBS MRCPCH
ST5 in Paediatrics, Whipps Cross University NHS Trust

Dr Arun J Baksi BSc (Hons) MBBS MRCP
SpR in Cardiology and G(I)M and Clinical Research Fellow, Imperial College
Healthcare NHS Trust and Imperial College London

Dr Thean Soon Chew BMedSci (Hons) MBChB (Hons) MRCP
Academic Clinical Fellow and Specialty Registrar in Gastroenterology,
University of Manchester and University College London

Dr Alexander J Clarke BSc (Hons) MBBS (Hons) MRCP (UK)
Specialist Registrar in Rheumatology and Wellcome Clinical Research
Training Fellow, Imperial College London

Dr Cordelia EM Coltart BSc (Hons) MBBS (Hons) MPH MRCP, DTM&H
Clinical Advisor to President of Royal College of Physicians in the Chief
Medical Officer's Clinical Advisors Scheme; ST4 Academic Clinical Fellow in
Infectious Diseases and Medical Microbiology, University College London
Hospitals NHS Trust and London School of Hygiene and Tropical Medicine

Dr David S Game MA BMBCh MRCP PhD FHEA
Consultant Nephrologist, Guy's and St Thomas' NHS Foundation Trust

Dr Charlotte RH Hedin BA BMBCh MRCP DTM&H
CORE Clinical Research Fellow in Gastroenterology, PhD student,
King's College London

Dr Susannah J Long MA MBBS MRCP
Specialist Registrar Geriatric Medicine and G(I)M, Hillingdon Hospital NHS
Trust and Clinical Research Fellow, Imperial College London

Dr Daniel JB Marks MBBS BSc (Hons) PhD MRCP
Academic Clinical Fellow in Translational Medicine, University College London

Dr Luke SP Moore MBChB MRCP DTM&H DipPH MSc
ST5 Specialty Registrar Infectious Diseases and Medical Microbiology,
Imperial College London

Dr Misha Moore BSc MBChB (Hons) DFFP MSc MRCOG
Registrar in Obstetrics and Gynaecology and Public Health, London Deanery

Dr Nuala R O'Shea BSc MBBS MRCP
Specialist Registrar in Gastroenterology, PhD student, Medical Research
Council Clinical Research Fellow, University College London

Dr Elspeth C Potton MA MBBchir MRCP
ST4 Academic Clinical Fellow in Respiratory Medicine, PhD student,
Wellcome Trust Clinical Research Fellow, University College London

Mr Gavin W Sewell BSc (Hons)
MB PhD student, University College London

Mr Joseph Shalhoub BSc (Hons) MBBS MRCS (Eng) FHEA
Clinical Research Fellow in Vascular Surgery, Imperial College London;
Specialty Registrar in General Surgery, North West Thames, London

Dr Andrew M Smith BSc (Hons) PhD
Senior Research Scientist, Department of Medicine, University College London

Professor Gordon W Stewart BSc MBChB MD FRCP
Professor of Experimental Medicine, University College London

Dr Stephen B Walsh MBBS MRCP PhD
Consultant Nephrologist, UCL Centre for Nephrology, Royal Free Hospital,
London

Dr M Justin S Zaman BSc MBBS MRCP MSc, PhD
NIHR Clinical Lecturer in Cardiology, University College London, UK

Foreword

Evidence-based medicine is the backdrop to medical education and practice, but the reality is that the evidence is often lacking. There is so much that we do not know about human physiology and variation between humans in both health and disease. Many of our current approaches to the prevention, diagnosis and management of illness are likely to appear primitive to future generations. A key quality of a good doctor is a sound understanding of the limits of his or her knowledge. In some cases asking a more experienced colleague or checking reference sources will provide the answer – but as often as not, the answer may be unknown. This is the starting point for research – and for the doctor imbued with a curious mind, there is no more exciting a career.

These are splendid times in which to be conducting medical research. It is possible to carry out research at a scale and depth that was inconceivable just a few years ago. Modern imaging techniques give both structural and functional insight into human physiology. High-throughput studies of DNA sequence and variation give access to the whole human genome and to the genomes of the multitude of organisms that inhabit and infect us. Proteomics and metabolomics, coupled with powerful microscopy, enable large-scale studies of the function of cells and organs. Animal models of disease can provide hugely informative approaches to exploring disease mechanisms both *in vivo* and *in vitro*. Large databases and longitudinal studies of healthy and diseased populations give access to the full range of human phenotypic variation, which can be related to differing environmental exposures and genetic variation. The possibilities of collaborating with chemists, physicists, mathematicians, computer scientists and engineers to develop new technologies for probing, preventing and treating disease are endless. The challenge to researchers assisted by such extraordinary tools for medical research is to identify and tackle important research questions and this is the key goal for any aspiring researcher.

The key characteristic of the clinical researcher is to conduct research that is informed by clinical training and exposure to the challenges and questions posed by the practice of clinical medicine. It is a demanding career because dual training is essential – in both clinical practice and research. Although dual training takes longer than single clinical or research training, the prospects for a fascinating career are unparalleled and with good mentorship the training period should be an enjoyable experience. It is crucial that first-class training opportunities are provided to new generations of clinical scientists in all areas of medicine. This means firstly attracting doctors into academic medicine by appropriate exposure to research as medical students and during junior postgraduate rotations. Secondly it means providing the environment and flexibility to enable the development of research skills in parallel with postgraduate clinical training in an integrated fashion. Thirdly there must be attractive career opportunities for high-quality trained clinical academic staff to enable them to establish independent careers as clinician scientists.

During the last few years in the UK a number of schemes have been developed specifically to address training in academic medicine – at all stages of the clinical career pathway, from foundation level, core and higher clinical training, to established academic positions as lecturer and senior lecturer. Navigating these pathways, and especially initial entry to academic medicine, can appear confusing and daunting. This new book provides an excellent guide to entering academic medicine via the different routes available in the UK, explaining the advantages and disadvantages, application processes, possibilities of research overseas and options for undertaking higher degrees or full-time research. Most importantly it demystifies the whole process to allow doctors (and medical students) to see how they may combine careers as clinicians and world-class scientists, or simply to get a flavour of academic medicine during clinical training. I hope that it will be useful to all those starting to explore careers in academic medicine.

Sir Mark Walport
Director of the Wellcome Trust
October 2010

Preface

"Discovery consists of seeing what everybody has seen and thinking what nobody has thought"

Albert Szent-Gyorgyi (1893–1986)

An academic medical career is not an easy one. In fact, it is probably the most challenging career path. The decision to enter academic medicine should not be made in haste. It should involve careful consideration about your personal motives and the decision needs to be as informed as possible. However, once you have made this choice you will undoubtedly embark on an exciting and fulfilling future – combing your clinical and academic passions to whatever extent you can.

To even consider making this choice you must seek advice from those in the speciality you want to enter or at least 'dip your toe' into it. This in itself can be difficult, although this is changing rapidly. There are still many in the academic field who are wary of offering advice to those seeking this as a career option. This may be fuelled by a sense of 'it was hard for me, so it should be hard for them' or a sense of cynicism and suspicion as to your reasons for wanting to take an academic path – 'it is only to boost your CV'. As a result, a mystical shroud has been cast over academic training, portraying an image of 'inaccessibility'.

This book though, together with the recent development of integrated academic training programmes, aims to remove the mystery and some of the hurdles surrounding an academic career pathway. Its credibility stems from its contributors and editors – all of whom have been involved in academic activities/careers and managing academic training – from the top levels to those just embarking. Their insight is crucial as first-hand knowledge and experience can help inform others. The book is split into sections to try and tackle crucial areas and challenges when entering and then staying in the academic field – from applications to interviews, funding and ethical considerations, through to common academic pitfalls and academic work overseas.

We have worked extremely hard to ensure the information contained within this book is relevant, accurate and as up to date as possible, to provide you with the best insider's guide to getting into academic medicine. The aim of this book is to inspire you to 'go for it', and to equip you with the tools required to remove any barriers that may slow your progress. Without doubt there will be those with differing opinions to the ones contained within this book, however we have endeavoured to provide the very best advice possible without of course knowing every individual's specific circumstances.

This book also aims to help you overcome such crucial hurdles as academic applications and interviews. Please remember however, that the example responses contained within this book should not be used as a template for your own responses – they are purely designed to give you a flavour of what is expected when you are at the stage of completing your own application! We hope you will use this book as a tool to assist and guide you through the potential routes into academic medicine and open your eyes to topics you may not have considered.

For those determined to pursue an academic career or tempted to see what it is like, we wish you all good luck!

PJS, SSN, JKG, JBL

Acknowledgements

We are very grateful to all the contributors for all their hard work in completing the chapters, and within a very tight timescale.

In addition, we offer our thanks to everyone at the RSM Press Ltd, as well as Hodder Arnold, who commissioned and supported this project – particularly Sarah Ogden and Caroline Makepeace.

PJS, SSN, JKS, JBL

Key to Icons

Beware

Example

Useful information

Pitfalls

Key points

Introduction to academic medicine

Introduction to academic medicine

Jasdeep K Gill
Sukhjinder S Nijjer
Jeremy B Levy
Philip J Smith

Medicine is a unique and dynamic vocation. Research and new discoveries form the foundation for the continuous evolution of, and changes in, medical practice. Academic medicine is the interface of high-quality patient care with exploration of basic questions of health and disease, prevention and treatment. All doctors therefore need to be aware how research can improve patient care and should have some understanding of the process. Ideally many should also undertake at least a period of research so they fully appreciate its challenges, excitement and potential. The drive to encourage research and support academia has been recognised by leaders in the National Health Service (NHS) as crucial to benefit patients and shape the future NHS. As part of this there are now more opportunities than ever for bright, motivated doctors to become academic clinicians, with proper research training and encouragement to remain in academia while maintaining patient contact. This whole book is aimed at encouraging young doctors (and medical students) to get into academic medicine, by explaining the routes available and the range of possibilities, exploring the pitfalls and suggesting solutions.

In 2005, the advent of Modernising Medical Careers (MMC) saw considerable reform to medical training. The lack of transparent career pathways, lack of flexibility between academic versus clinical training, and lack of structured posts once training had been completed were all highlighted as obstacles within academic medicine. A report produced by MMC and the UK Clinical Research Collaboration (UKCRC), known as the *Walport Report*, addressed many of these issues by generating recommendations for the training of future researchers and educators, and has been implemented to a significant degree by the UK Department of Health.

What is research and why do it?

Both research and audit are important undertakings for doctors in training but are very different (in fact this is a popular question at interviews for academic training). Audit is a cyclical process whereby current practice is compared with established or aspirational guidelines, or 'gold standards'. It is a means of quality assurance, prompts improvements in service and calls for re-audit to 'close the loop' by confirming that changes made have had positive impacts on provision of care or patient outcomes. Audit should be a routine part of clinical life.

Research encompasses the activities that offer evidence upon which these standards can be set, and answers fundamental questions about cause and consequence. These intellectual activities hope eventually in clinical medicine to elucidate new diagnostic and therapeutic strategies. Research is a spectrum from molecular and cellular laboratory exploration through to clinical implementation. The successful shift from bench to bedside is often termed 'translational research'; it hopes to allow prompt changes to be made to practice for the benefit of patients.

Why undertake a period of research? Certainly benefits accrue to trainees themselves, the wider medical community, future employers and of course patients. Knowledge will be gained by all in some form or another. Trainees who enjoyed previous exposure to research are encouraged to pursue this further. They have the opportunity to further their own understanding in a specific field, being able to add to currently available knowledge, which can be highly rewarding. Clinician scientists can become experts in an (admittedly often small) area, which is also personally satisfying but can drive up standards more widely; having this 'niche' will also demonstrate a commitment to a speciality and improve your 'saleability' when applying for future posts.

Individuals will acquire transferable skills, such as statistical knowledge, critical appraisal of literature (which facilitates the practice of evidence-based medicine), problem solving and 'thinking outside box', time management (the art of juggling), self-motivation, discipline and being a 'self-starter'. Public speaking and presentation skills will be improved and the ability to take an idea, implement a project and take it through to completion and wider dissemination. Of course you might have caught the bug at university and aspire to become the Professor of Medicine or Surgery or Primary Care and should not be put off the attempt.

Choosing academic medicine

Your decision to enter academic medicine can be as difficult as choosing to enter medical school or choosing your speciality. Academic medicine offers you a unique opportunity to use your experience and research to shape future practice. Having a transparent and structured pathway to your academic career certainly helps. However, you will undoubtedly have several more hurdles to negotiate successfully before starting your research. The practicalities of applying, obtaining funding and identifying a supervisor are only a few of the encounters ahead of you. Therefore it is important that you carefully consider your decision to enter academic medicine. Start discussing your thoughts with colleagues and potential supervisors *early*. Try to establish from your discussions if you see yourself in academic medicine, and see if you can acquire an academic mentor. However, beware that one person's experience can be very different from that of another. Be honest with yourself about your abilities.

Beware!
- Beware of the widely varied experiences of trainees within academic medicine
- Be honest with yourself about your skills and abilities

If you have identified a particular area of interest, you should try to undertake some 'shadowing' or organise meetings with supervisors to enable you to find out more about this. You should enquire about potential projects, current research in that area, future niches for your potential work and how it may relate to your future career.

You should also discuss your thoughts and plans with family. You may have financial, personal or geographical considerations that need to be taken into account. You will need to develop a suitable balance between your research, clinical commitments and personal life. This can sometimes be harder to achieve than you first expect. Having support from colleagues and family goes a long way in your success.

Walport Report: training medical researchers and educators of the future

This report was specifically produced to improve the career structures for academics in medicine (and dentistry). It was generated by the Academic Careers Sub-Committee of the UKCRC and MMC and was chaired by the Director of the Wellcome Trust, Sir Mark Walport. Previous reports from many bodies had highlighted difficulties encountered by aspiring academics and growing concerns over the reducing numbers entering academia in several medical and surgical specialities. The Academic Careers Sub-Committee's developed sustainable solutions to the obstacles and the final *Walport Report* mapped out new pathways to aid junior doctors to pursue a career in academic medicine. The recommendations from this report focussed on four key milestones in a clinician's career (medical school, foundation programme, specialist training and established consultant/GP: see Boxes 1.1–1.6) and the recommendations have in the most part been implemented.

Box 1.1 Medical school#

- Medical students must be informed of careers in academic medicine and how to pursue them
- Maintain the opportunity to undertake an intercalated BSc degree or equivalent
- Use appropriate programmes within the undergraduate curriculum, such as special study modules to allow opportunity for exploring academia
- Develop programmes for obtaining higher qualifications in education

Box 1.2 Foundation programme#

- Offer opportunities for an integrated academic foundation year 2 (F2) programme either with academic activities incorporated throughout the year or a 4-month academic block within the F2 year
- A 2-year integrated academic foundation programme, particularly targeting MB-PhD graduates

Box 1.3 Specialist training#

- Develop competitive dedicated and structured academic training programmes at two levels, namely academic clinical fellowships (ACFs) leading to a training fellowship and higher degree with external funding; clinical lectureships (CLs) leading to the certificate of completion of training (CCT) and postdoctoral opportunities
- National competition to gain entry onto these programmes
- A variety of entry points should exist that are open to trainees who wish to enter the academic pathway later during their clinical pathway
- A national training number (academic) (NTN(A)) given upon successful entry
- Funding of research should not be restricted to award only those with an NTN(A)
- Exit from the academic training programme to return to usual clinical training can be undertaken at any point providing satisfactory joint academic and clinical appraisals
- Actively develop programmes in particular specialties that have undergone a decline in academic activity

Box 1.4 Academic GP specialist training#

- Create 2-year academic posts, with 50% clinical and 50% academic time
- Entry to these posts should be available during and after completion of the vocational training scheme
- Create 1-year funding scheme to give salary support for GPs who wish to prepare an application for postdoctoral fellowship
- No distinction in pay rates between senior academic versus clinical GPs

---

Box 1.5 Trainees taking a career break#

- Develop a mentoring scheme to support trainees prior to and after a career break
- Develop 're-entry' programmes for trainees after extended career breaks

---

Box 1.6 Consultant/GP#

- Create senior lectureship posts to accommodate the new generation of trained clinical academics ('new blood' senior lectureships)
- Allow further clinical training depending on career requirements
- Pay parity must exist between clinical academics and their NHS counterparts

---

A day in the life of an academic

Each speciality is different and each day is diverse with an assortment of ups and downs. Depending on the stage within your research, you will have different goals, tasks, responsibilities and expectations. Therefore of course a 'typical day' does not really exist. To give you an idea and some appreciation of what may lie ahead we have included some examples in our Ask the expert boxes.

Ask the expert

A day in the life of Surgical Research Fellow, Mr Joseph Shalhoub, doing laboratory-based research

6.15am	Get up, jot down a few ideas and send a few emails
7.00am	Breakfast
7.30am	Leave home
7.45am	Arrive at work and pop up to the intensive-care unit (ITU) to check on a postoperative patient who was unstable overnight, as I was on call last night
8.00am	Handover
8.10am	Meet with the academic F2, who I am supervising, over coffee to discuss his progress and the week's plan
8.30am	Start immunohistochemical staining of cryosectioned human carotid plaque tissue. An Undergraduate Research Opportunities Programme student is observing the technique. This is a multiple-step process, interspersed with numerous short breaks. These are spent teaching the student, popping to my supervisors' offices or on my laptop:

- Writing or reviewing a paper
- Writing or correcting thesis chapters
- Emailing
- Planning future experiments

#**Boxes 1.1–1.6** Recommendations at clinician career milestones as given in *Walport Report*.

- Writing grant applications
- Completing ethics forms or amendments
- Submitting abstracts for conferences
- Preparing a PowerPoint exhibit for a forthcoming presentation
- Collecting tissue specimens from theatre

1.00pm	Lunch at my desk
1.20pm	Analyse data from a recent multi-analyte profiling experiment
2.30pm	Return to experiment
6.00pm	Finish experiment and debrief with student
6.30pm	Return to research fellows' room to meet with colleague about a prospective clinical study on stroke prediction in carotid stenosis that we are running, and other projects
8.00pm	Leave for home, have dinner with wife in front of TV, usually re-runs of *Friends*
10.00pm	Reply to emails and read in bed
10.30pm	Lights out

Ask the expert

A day in the life of Gastroenterology Academic Clinical Fellow, Dr Philip Smith, doing laboratory-based research involved collection of clinical samples from patients

6.00am	Wake up, get changed, say goodbye to the 'missus'!
6.10am	Cycle to work
6.40am	Arrive at work, have a shower
7.00am	Sort through emails, prepare final part of presentation, ensure culture medium warmed up in incubator
8.00am	Prepare cultured cells and plan the rest of this morning's experiments
8.30am	Meet academic supervisor to plan current and forthcoming research direction
9.30am	Stimulate the cultured cells and prepare for RNA purification
11.30am	Complete RNA purification and start analysing data from last experiment
12.30am	Present at Grand round (change pants afterwards!)
1.30pm	Eat lunch on way to Endoscopy list
1.45pm	Start Endoscopy list – collecting intestinal biopsies for research at the same time
3.15pm	Finish Endoscopy list and head back to laboratory
3.30pm	Store intestinal biopsies in –70°C freezer and update patient database
4.00pm	Start teaching core medical trainees in preparation for MRCP(UK) Part 2 Clinical Examination (PACES) examination
5.30pm	Cycle home
8.00pm	Sit down for dinner, catch up on the day's events, relax in front of TV and speak to the family
9.00pm	Write up a few outstanding publications unrelated to current research
10.30pm	Answer any outstanding emails
11.00pm	Off to sleep – absolutely shattered!

■ Further reading

Clinical Academic Medicine: The way forward. A report from the Forum on Academic Medicine. Forum on Academic Medicine (November 2004)

Clinical academic staffing levels in UK medical and dental schools. The Council of Medical Schools and the Council of Deans of Dental Schools (May 2004)

Developing and sustaining a world class workforce of educators and researchers in health and social care: StLaR HR Plan Project Phase II Strategic Report. The Strategic Learning and Research Advisory Group (August 2004)

Medically and dentally qualified academic staff: Recommendations for training the researchers and educators of the future. Report of the Academic Careers Sub-Committee of Modernising Medical Careers and the UK Clinical Research Collaboration (March 2005)

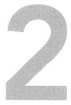

Pathways into academic medicine

Charlotte RH Hedin

Academic medicine offers a unique position at the interface between basic science and clinical practice. No profession is better placed to facilitate translational research. Academic qualifications will make you more competitive and clinical academics often have more freedom to devise their own job plans. Having an academic slant to your career and CV will improve your employment prospects, as well as providing intellectual stimulation and the opportunity to follow your own ideas. You also have the chance to travel and attend international meetings. With constant restructuring of the NHS having an academic interest can bring funding for your post and help secure employment. For these reasons, and many more, doctors are often attracted to it. However, deciding when the time is right for you to enter academic medicine can be difficult. In this and the next chapter we will explore various routes into academic medicine and the different points in medical careers this can happen.

▧ When to enter academic medicine

The optimal time to enter academic medicine depends on *you*. Your academic career could start as early as medical school, or even before. Opportunities are available during foundation programme training or speciality training, in the gaps between or at most stages within your career. When and how you choose to enter will be heavily influenced by your speciality, your research interests, family and other commitments as well as the opportunities available and serendipity. Before entering academic medicine, you should discuss your plans openly with colleagues, family members and most importantly potential supervisors.

Your route into academic medicine will depend upon when you decide that academia is for you. The pathway you follow subsequently will be determined by the timing of your entry and your career aspirations. It is ideal to have a medium-term plan, which you should discuss with an academic mentor. The *Walport Report*, in an attempt to rejuvenate academic medicine in the UK and optimise academic and clinical training, suggested the notion of an integrated academic training path (Figure 2.1). Academic posts would be created at foundation level and during specialist training to encourage more clinicians to take up research training fellowships and ultimately clinical lectureships (CLs) and aim for senior lecturer and professorial posts. Such posts have been created. However this is not the only route into academic medicine, and although a few trainees may progress from an academic foundation post, into an ACF post, a PhD programme and then becoming a clinical lecturer, this is in fact quite rare. Entry (and exit) can occur at many stages.

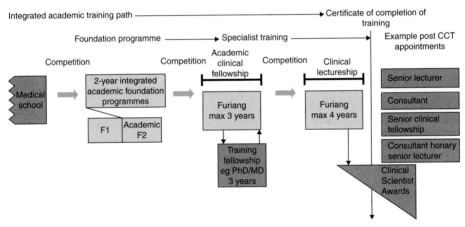

Figure 2.1 Integrated academic training path. Reproduced from the Foundation Programme website

Key points

- Think about where you see yourself and your career in 5–10 years' time and even beyond that!
- Remember to consider personal and financial issues as well as what suits your speciality
- Do not be too rigid with your plan – you may find yourself at the right place at the right time and take up an opportunity you weren't expecting
- Be open and talk about your plans to enter academic medicine and seek advice from colleagues, family members, supervisors and ideally an academic mentor

Medical school or before

You may have already done or want to consider an undergraduate or postgraduate degree before you enter medical school. Alternatively many medical schools either award undergraduate degrees as part of their (usually 6-year) medical training programme or you can opt to do an *intercalated* BSC. Opinions differ over the value of degrees awarded simply as part of a 6-year programme, versus those who compete with peers to undertake a limited number of intercalated degrees. Your options may be limited by your medical school, but some look favourably at requests to undertake an intercalated BSc at another university. Funding, however, may be an issue. Either option should provide you with a fantastic opportunity to get some research under your belt, a flavour of academic medicine and potentially some publications. Try to submit at least one abstract and enter your research project for prizes or even a national or international conference. Be enthusiastic and your supervisor will ensure your efforts are rewarded. All of this will hugely enhance your CV, may excite and stimulate you, and will score valuable points during any shortlisting when you apply for any post after qualifying. Such degrees are especially important when applying for ACF posts or research training fellowships. The classification of the degree (e.g. 1st, 2.1, 2.2) is also important with more kudos given to better degrees and more points on an application form.

There are also MD PhD programmes that will allow you to complete an undergraduate medical degree and PhD during your medical training. These are rare in the UK, and although allowing you to continue research after a BSc to a high level can have major disadvantages.

Advantages

★ Early experience of research will allow you to develop your academic interests to complement your entire clinical career.
★ Research is often paid less, so doing full-time research early in your career when your financial and family commitments may be lower can be an advantage.
★ Similarly earlier in your career you may be more likely to have the freedom to move to the institution or country where the departmental interests match yours, allowing you to take advantage of a wider range of opportunities.
★ In some instances you may make contacts with researchers in the university during your medical training and it can be valuable to build upon this relationship by pursuing a postgraduate degree during or after medical school.
★ Delaying entry to medical school such that you are more mature and experienced when you start clinical training may also be an advantage.
★ A degree or PhD, particularly in biomedical areas, will clearly be an advantageous platform from which to launch both your clinical and academic career.

⋆ Undertaking a PhD during your undergraduate clinical training is less open to distractions of clinical work and you may be more productive academically.

Disadvantages

⋆ You will be older than your peers at medical school and going back to a fully taught course may feel retrograde when you are already used to greater intellectual freedom.
⋆ Before you have had any real clinical exposure it may be difficult to predict where your clinical interests will lie and you may find your PhD topic is not relevant to final chosen speciality. This matters less if it is in a basic science, and in the end matters little if you can use your intellectual abilities and acquired translational skills.
⋆ Prolonging your undergraduate training will mean you are likely to leave university with greater debts. In addition, although going into research from a clinical job represents a big drop in salary, you are likely to be paid even less as a PhD student without a medical degree.
⋆ If your research was stellar it is very difficult to keep it going after completing a PhD and re-entering clinical undergraduate medical training and then early postgraduate training.

Foundation years

Fully integrated 1- or 2-year 'academic' foundation year placements, including clinical time and research or teaching opportunities, based in a single institution (usually) are available and extremely highly sought after. These are competitively awarded when you apply to the Foundation programme separately and in advance of the routine foundation programme selection process. On your application form you will need to score highly, and evidence of previous research of any kind and the *potential* to do research is essential, together with a good degree and/or prizes at university or subsequently. There are several different models of academic foundation programmes around the UK and in different deaneries and universities. Some leave the F1 year as a purely clinical year and concentrate the academic activities into the F2 year, whilst others integrate this into both years. Some offer teaching as the academic component with training in teaching during the period. The academic component might be offered as a 4-month block or as a day release each week. In some academic primary care programmes the time can be fully integrated with time in general practice or public health departments. There are likely to be overarching training programmes or courses covering teaching skills, ethics, academic careers guidance etc. The aim of such programmes is not to give enough time to produce world-shattering research (impossible in 4 months of course) but to give a flavour of academic medicine so that incumbents can decide whether to pursue a PhD, for example via the ACF route.

It is crucial to use the time available to you in such posts well and plan ahead very carefully. Some trainees have found it difficult to be productive in the 4-month secondment. Some have also abused the time and used it for lounging, simply because the pace is slower than while in clinical ward posts. Some departments have a clear structured programme whereas others may use the foundation doctor as an 'extra pair of hands' (avoid such posts!). Furthermore, it is exceptionally difficult to do original research in such a time frame. Therefore you must approach your academic supervisor at the earliest opportunity, even before you begin the foundation programme, so you can start lining up a research project, start reading and understanding the area of research. It may be that you continue the research project in some way throughout the year in your spare time. It is certainly possible to achieve good publications during this time, or at the least to get your name on an abstract or presentation at a national meeting, to experience what academic medicine is about, and to be enthused by academic physicians around you and those doing their PhDs.

Your output from an academic foundation programme will really depend on what you put into it. Use the time well and you can set up a healthy academic career. Even those who do not enter a specific academic programme, can still approach supervisors during their foundation programme and try to gain some research experience. For example you could help collect data for your registrar's PhD project or help log data for your department's registry database and analyse it. From small beginnings it's certainly possible to gain publications and excellent (although of course limited) experience in research.

Advantages

* Demonstrating your academic interest early is an advantage in itself and is the ideal basis on which to build your application for an ACF.
* Having first-hand experience of the discipline of research whether that be laboratory based or clinical will give your funding applications a more authoritative tone (or help you decide academic medicine is not for you!).
* Maintaining contact with academic departments throughout your training will ensure you are aware of research opportunities as they arise.
* Those who take part in research early are more likely to have *more* publications than those similarly qualified but who enter research later – simply being associated with a research department will lead to publication opportunities and the chance to be part of other people's work.

Disadvantages

* At this early stage in your career you may be more enthused by opportunities for clinical exposure and may therefore not want to devote time to research.
* You may feel that taking time out at this stage risks losing those clinical skills that you are only just getting to grips with.
* You will in fact need to work doubly hard during your clinical periods as your patient exposure time is less and you will still need to meet all the

same clinical competencies as your colleagues. This is crucial since failing to show clinical competence will mean repeating time in the foundation years.
* Many trainees at this level are not sure which speciality they want to follow. You may risk finding that your clinical interests develop in a different direction from your early research projects. However this is *not* a major disadvantage at all since research skills are transferable and working in several areas will broaden your scientific horizons.
* Sometimes these posts can be less well planned than they should be. Therefore you should ask about the programme and try to ensure that your project is clearly defined and tailored to fit into the 4-month slot. Talk to the academic programme lead and your academic supervisors early and well before you start.

Academic clinical fellowship

These are 3-year speciality training posts that incorporate academic training into clinical training, aiming to prepare you for a full-time research training fellowship. You will spend 75% of the time in clinical training and 25% in research or training in medical education. During the 3 years in the ACF post, or 4 years for general practice speciality trainees, you would be expected to work towards securing doctoral (research) training fellowship funding, allowing you then to spend a further 3 years in full-time research, completing an MD or PhD before rejoining the training scheme. ACF posts are generally at ST3 level in medical and surgical specialties, but may be at ST1 level in programmes with 'run-through' training such as paediatrics or public health. This varies around the UK by deanery and the hosting university.

Once you have completed the 3-year period the ACF status will end and you will need to apply for a CL or other post-doctoral post (after the PhD) in order to continue your academic career. Alternatively, you can return to your clinical programme and pursue this until you reach CCT stage. ACF posts are covered in detail in Chapter 3.

Similar schemes to the ACF exist in Scotland, supervised by the Chief Scientist Office (www.cso.scot.nhs.uk). In Wales, the Wales Clinical Academic Track (WCAT) is an 8-year scheme including 3-year PhD and period of clinical training as well as dedicated academic time in the later years of the scheme.

For GP speciality trainees there is a similar scheme run by the National Institute of Health School for Primary Care Research, which allows an extension of GP training by 1 year to allow academic training and clinical training to be combined. In many of these posts you are encouraged to study for an MSc in Primary Care or Medical Science whilst also supporting development of your fellowship application. For GPs who are already fully qualified there are National Institute of Health in Practice Fellowships.

Advantages

* ACFs and their equivalents are usually very well supported and will give you a competitive advantage in putting together a more convincing research fellowship application.
* Having dedicated time available to get some pilot data, or learn some research skills is invaluable.
* Many offer taught training in specific academic skills such as constructing a funding application and in research ethics.
* Often you will carry out research (e.g. pilot studies) during the ACF that can inform and improve the design of your higher-degree project.
* Having completed a significant amount of your clinical training you may feel more confident to leave or reduce clinical work at this stage without risking losing essential skills that you have worked hard to acquire.
* Many doctors who have children or other commitments reduce their clinical workload during this phase of their career and the enhanced flexibility in research may allow you to fit your work around other demands.

Disadvantages

* The 75% clinical and 25% research ratio can mean that research time is squeezed – especially as your research is competing with very busy clinical jobs.
* You are likely to spend a series of short periods (i.e. 3 months per year) in research, which can be disruptive.
* Some programmes have an unusual approach of giving you a 'day a week' of research, which is much harder to use constructively.
* Taking career breaks such as maternity leave will decrease the momentum of your research career.

The contacts you make and publications you produce during these early years will be the springboard from which you will launch your academic career so you may wish to consider delaying career breaks until the final part of your training or at consultant level.

■ Out-of-programme experiences

It is certainly possible to undertake a period of clinical research without the prelude of a defined clinical academic post like an ACF. This was the traditional route into academic medicine before ACF posts were created. It is the route your supervisors will have followed.

Regardless of whether you have used an ACF post or your spare time to win a research fellowship or other funded period of research, you will have to have a national training number (NTN) and have completed your ST1 (or 3) year (depending on speciality). In order to take the time out of clinical training to do the research you must apply for an out-of-programme (OOP) period. This is a formal break in your clinical training programme to allow you to do other activities. If you do not take such a break for 2–3 years you cannot achieve any significant academic work or research training. Four types of OOP exist in the *Fact* box.

> **Useful information**
>
> 1 Out of programme for experience (OOPE).
> 2 Out of programme for training (OOPT).
> 3 Out of programme for a career break (OOPC).
> 4 Out of programme for research (OOPR).

If you are able to secure funding for a doctoral research fellowship then you can apply to your deanery for OOPR to cover the duration of this degree, usually up to 3 years, allowing you to retain your NTN and re-enter the training programme when you have completed the degree. If your proposed research time is between training programmes, e.g. between core medicine and higher medical training (after CT2) or between foundation and core training, then you do not need to apply for OOPR since you are not actually within a training programme.

Advantages

* By avoiding splitting your time between clinical and research during your speciality training you will gain more clinical experience prior to entering research.
* Research conducted at this stage in your career will be within the speciality that you have already chosen.
* Your research may well define your career so knowing what you want your final career destination to be when choosing your project for your thesis is a definite advantage.
* Many specialities include research registrars into the out-of-hours on-call rota (e.g. surgery, gastroenterology, cardiology, neurology, oncology and many more) allowing you to supplement your income by being on call. This may allow you to avoid a large drop in salary during full-time research.

Disadvantages

* You cannot use OOPR to plan your research, thus if you don't have an ACF post you will have to work at evenings and weekends to prepare for the research time. The OOPR can only be started when research funding/ a fellowship has become available. This will undoubtedly place a strain on you, though it is the 'original' way to plan your PhD/MD.
* Starting research at this stage (during higher training) means it will be a long time since you were last in a laboratory or using other research skills, and you may find yourself relearning skills you have not used since medical school.
* You will have been getting used to a degree of seniority and will have been valued in your clinical job. Becoming a PhD student can feel like going back

to foundation level – you may find yourself having to ask your research colleagues about simple things.

* Going into research from a clinical job will mean the potential drop in salary is more acute – and this will be at a time when you may have acquired more commitments, including a mortgage and family.

Post-doctoral research

Once you have completed your doctoral degree there are a range of pathways to follow. Some people are satisfied that they have achieved their goal of producing a piece of original research, and may wish to focus on clinical activities either within the NHS or private practice. Some may wish to devote more time to their family and other outside interests and return to clinical medicine without pursuing academic activities further. You will of course need to complete your clinical training unless you decide to leave clinical medicine permanently.

Alternatively you may go on to take up a clinical post that includes protected research or teaching time. If you are appointed in a clinical post with links to an active university department you may be able to collaborate with scientists to contribute to translational research. The posts providing most protected research time are CLs (see Chapter 3), in which 50% of your time can be used to continue and elaborate on your research. Alternatively you may be able to inspire and supervise your junior staff to carry out clinical projects within your NHS practice.

If you intend to develop yourself as a leader in clinical academia, there are specific posts and funding schemes that will allow you to do this. These include the Postdoctoral Training Fellowships for MB/PhD graduates offered by the MRC and the National Institute of Health Research Clinical Lectureships. These allow you to combine completing clinical training at registrar level with research. In Scotland there are CSO Fellowships – post-doctoral posts that are equivalent to CLs in England. In addition Wellcome Trust Intermediate Clinical Fellowships are aimed at those who have obtained a higher degree and have or are about to finish their clinical training but have not yet secured a permanent (consultant level) post. The tenure is between 4 and 5 years depending on how much clinical training you need to complete. Beyond these there are the Clinician Scientist Fellowships and Clinician Scientist awards (at consultant level).

Balancing academic medicine

Many clinical academics can feel they have two full-time jobs rather than one split equally! You will be under great pressure from both clinical medicine and academia making demands on you, for example for grant applications, publications, outpatient clinic and operative waiting targets, infection control and attracting PhD students. You must manage your time very carefully and be sure not to degrade the quality of your work by taking on too much.

Protect your research time. This is facilitated by the new, more structured clinical academic career path, such as entering an ACF. However at all levels you will need to ensure that you negotiate adequate academic time with your NHS employer, and remember it works both ways.

Beware!
- Beware of running out of time – you don't have as long as you think!
- Things can get very stressful if you don't plan or keep on top of your work

You will have less clinical exposure during training than your full-time clinical colleagues and you need to ensure that your training goals are clear and that you make sure you have enough of the relevant clinical exposure to achieve these goals. A common trap is re-entering full-time clinical training without having completed writing your doctoral thesis. Attempting to write a complex, lengthy academic document in your 'spare time' can be a miserable undertaking and unfortunately sometimes leads to the thesis never being completed or submitted. In order to avoid the disaster of non-submission you will have to endure many weekends and evenings of writing-up on top of your full-time clinical job. Prevent this by planning the last few months of your research time carefully to allow yourself to complete the majority, or better still, your entire thesis before returning to clinical training.

Key points
- Clinical–research balance
  - Start early so you have enough time to write and secure your grant
  - Protect your research time
  - Complete your thesis and publications *during* your research time
- Research–life balance
  - See it in perspective
  - Tackle the research in manageable 'bite size' sections, so you don't become overwhelmed and have sleepless nights
  - If you have other commitments or choose to do any locum shifts, plan ahead and don't let it impede your research

Taking time out from research

Maternity leave

Research can be the best and worst time to take maternity leave, or rather research is a very bad time from which to take maternity leave but often a good time to go back to work from it. During a maternity leave period your research may become out of date and most projects will need tweaking at the very least, or sometimes need major re-writing if you are unlucky when you return to work.

You may lose some research skills, or lose track of projects. It can be an advantage however, as you may be able to make changes in the light of your experience of research work generally and of your project specifically, and other developments more widely. An opportunity to re-evaluate what you are doing may improve your project. In contrast to a clinical job where apart from a little rustiness, a return to work will be fairly seamless, in research you may no longer be current and things in your field or your department may have moved on significantly since you were last there. Once you return to work you will experience what will initially seem like the unimaginably impossible task that all working mothers (and to some extent fathers) face of balancing family and work life. It is hard to get this balance right in any workplace but in research, particularly non-clinical research, you have much greater flexibility to tailor this around your family's needs. Although research cannot be done just 9–5, it is certainly possible to arrange laboratory or office work around childcare more easily often than clinical work with on-call commitments, sick patients and busy wards. In terms of practicalities of maternity leave pay, it is important that a research post, if possible, is funded to maintain your NHS terms of employment, and you should check this carefully with your HR department. Without this your accrued maternity rights may be in jeopardy.

There are efforts to improve the recruitment and retention of women in academic medicine. Data collected by the Medical Schools Council show that the number of women working in clinical academia decreases at each grade of the academic career ladder, with only 11% of professorial staff in medicine being female, compared to 36% at clinical lecturer level. Given that the proportion of women entrants to medical school each year has been over 50% since around 1996, this has raised concerns that clinical academia will suffer if more women are not attracted to this type of post. Most employers should therefore be keen to facilitate the progression of women through clinical academia. Clinical academia is a more complex career path than a pure clinical career, but the juggling act is much more difficult with yet another full-time job thrown in. Even with a supportive academic department it may be difficult to maintain your career momentum if you are going to take on much of the day-to-day responsibility of caring for your children.

Beware!

Maternity leave pitfalls

1 Check your entitlement to maternity leave and pay (ideally before you get pregnant!). For those in a NHS-based post (e.g. ACF) you will be a trust employee and therefore entitled to the NHS maternity pay. Similarly if you are classed as a university staff member you will be eligible for the university's maternity pay scheme. CLs are generally employed by a university. If you are currently paid from a fellowship by for example a charity (e.g. during a PhD), you may not be covered by either of these

and there are unlikely to be funds in your grant to cover maternity pay. Discuss directly with the body funding your research what arrangements are available.

2 For most jobs you have to have been in continuous employment in your current post for a specified amount of time before you are eligible to claim for maternity pay. In most instances moving from NHS to a university post or vice versa is not considered a new post and you can maintain your continuous employment record, but it is worth checking.

3 Beware the temptation to promise your supervisors that you will finish that grant application/write up your thesis/submit that *Nature* paper whilst on maternity leave. Having lots of on-call experience, you may think you know about being up all night, but remember that with a baby no one gives you the day off the next day to sleep and you're on call for baby every night for weeks, months… years. Babies are nothing if not relentless!

Paternity leave

You will be entitled to the standard 2 weeks paternity leave and if you are fully employed either by an NHS trust or a university – this is statutory. If you have a sympathetic supervisor paternity leave is much easier to coordinate than maternity leave for obvious reasons. However, if you are doing a PhD funded by a grant in your supervisor's name then it is at his or her discretion. There are rumours of supervisors who do not believe in annual leave during PhDs, so beware! A clear advantage of academic life over clinical work is that you can take leave at short notice without having to worry about that on-call or whether clinic is covered.

Beware!

Paternity leave pitfalls

1 You will have months to plan so try and make sure that you are not running a set of critical experiments around the time of delivery (remember babies come both early and late) so use your common sense.

2 Beware planning to supplement your salary with night shifts whilst also doing full-time research and looking after the kids: it is likely that one will take a backseat and this is usually the research.

3 In many ways having children whilst in academia is easier than clinical work in that the on-calls are either non-existent or from home and there are fewer 5.00pm emergencies such as presented by the sick ward patient or disastrous clinic. However you will need to plan your time carefully if you want to ensure that you can be at home to help out or pick the kids up from the childminder.

4 Do not underestimate how much time the new arrival in your life will take up. It is likely that those productive late evening sessions when everyone else in the lab had gone home and you had time to write in peace will instead be taken up with nappies, bath time and keeping your partner sane.

Key points for clinical academic parents

1 Forget about defining the perfect balance between work and family! In academic medicine and in families your priorities change from week to week – see it as dynamic imbalance and be prepared to juggle.
2 Decide what you really want to do. You can't do academic work, clinical work, teaching, run the medical school, have a lucrative private practice and expect to have your kids be able to recognise you. Drop some of the things you do and prioritise your goals. Don't waste time doing things that won't help you reach those goals. Cut out anything that does not add to your career to free up more family time.
3 You will need help. Accept any and all help offered and if you can afford it buy more help. Most clinical academics cite support from their spouse as a key to their success but it is harder if you both have challenging careers or if you are a single parent. Grandparents are the most valuable resource if they are willing to help and even more so if they live close by. Accept that day care will be a big part of your kids' life so invest in it.
4 Take advantage of the flexibility that research affords you. Unlike your dedicated childless colleagues, you may have to leave right on the dot of five to pick your kids up from childcare – but in contrast to clinical work much of your academic work can be done at home at 9.00pm once your kids are in bed. You can also pop into the lab to finish your experiment at the weekend, leaving your kids with the other parent or a grandparent. However do not underestimate the exhaustion factor: switching on the laptop at 9.00pm after a long day might not be quite as attractive an option as you originally hoped.

Flexible training

The most common reason to reduce your working hours is being a parent of young children. This is also given highest priority when determining who is eligible for 'less-than full-time' work, along with those who want to care for sick or dependent relatives and those who are unable, for health reasons, to work full time. Flexible training status may also be granted to doctors wishing to train part time, while in other paid or unpaid employment for the remainder of the week and those wishing to train part time in order to follow non-medical interests, for example, undertake sporting or musical activity. In these cases you will need to have a strong case to persuade your deanery to give you flexible training status, such as playing or competing at national or even international level. In such cases funding is available for doctors in clinical training posts. Flexible training will not be granted for you to undertake research by a deanery. If you want to return or take up research less than full time you will need to raise this with the funding body and your supervisor to see if it is at all possible, and it is not a right. Check carefully.

> **Pitfalls**
>
> **Flexible training pitfalls**
>
> 1 Examine your proposed job plan carefully. Clinical and academic work are both very demanding on your time and it may be all too easy to end up doing the same amount of work but getting paid less. In reality working less than full time and continuing clinical and academic work is very difficult.
> 2 Defend your training opportunities. Service commitments often squeeze the time available for training and this may be harder to resist when the time you are at work is limited.
> 3 Training as an academic alongside your clinical training prolongs the time it takes to reach consultant level. Adding flexible training to this will stretch out your training even further. You may join the ranks of those who have been a registrar for a decade or more.
> 4 Downsize your goals. It is unrealistic to expect that you can achieve as much working part time as you can working full time. Be selective about what you focus on and be prepared to let some things go. It is better to do fewer things well than spread yourself too thinly.

Summary

As a clinical academic your career structure will be more complex in comparison to a pure clinical job. The necessity to balance and manage your career is therefore greater. However, you will also have more independence to develop your interests and greater flexibility to shape these to fit your personal circumstances. There are probably as many pathways through academic medicine as there are clinical academics.

Acknowledgements

The author wishes to thank CORE for financial support in the form of a clinical fellowship and Dr Gareth Parkes for the section on paternity leave.

Further reading

Johansen KL. Women in nephrology: one mother's strategies for success in academic medicine. *Kidney Int* 2008;74:401–2

Medical Schools Council. *Women in Clinical Academia: Attracting and Developing the Medical and Dental Workforce of the Future.* Aldridge Press, 2007

Routes into academic medicine

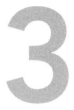

The ACF, CL and alternative routes

Elspeth C Potton
Nuala O'Shea

Academic clinical fellowships (ACFs) and clinical lectureships (CLs) were novel posts created to address the shortage of senior medical academics in the UK and to try and establish an integrated academic training programme encouraging more people to take up academic careers. Prior to this there was no formally recognised training scheme for academic medicine to ensure that high-quality individuals were recruited, trained and then retained to work within NHS trusts and associated universities. These changes were the result of the implementation of the *Walport Report*. In this chapter we will discuss some of the benefits of these training posts, how to apply, how to get the most out of the jobs and the roles of some research organisations. Later in the chapter we will consider alternative routes for entering research separate from the ACF system, which prior to the *Walport Report* were seen as 'traditional routes'. Your supervisors will likely have used the traditional route, and there are still alternative routes into academic medicine.

Academic clinical fellowships

These are 3-year training posts that are managed jointly by the deanery, university and allied NHS trust. Recruitment can be very competitive and is managed either locally by a deanery and university or sometimes nationally for the smaller specialities. The posts are available at ST3 level usually in medical and surgical specialties, but can be at ST1 level in run-through specialties such as paediatrics or public health. This though can vary by deanery, university and specific post or training scheme. In these posts you are usually employed by the NHS trust but have an honorary contract with the university medical school. Your time is split 75% clinical training and 25% academic training but the precise arrangement can vary from post to post. Furthermore, how the academic time is spread across the year (or even 3 years) can also vary: some provide a fixed period of 3 months in a year, others may give you a day a week, others may allow 6 months over a 2-year period in one block.

The principle advantage of an ACF post is that you have paid time available to develop a research idea, seek funding and write a grant application for a PhD. You can use the time to explore research options. For example you might use the first 3 months to spend time in three different research groups to determine which area interests you most, and the second block to start experiments in the chosen area and writing a fellowship application. The aim is to apply successfully for a research training fellowship (RTF) to complete a PhD. In some cases an MD will be accepted. When you enter your training fellowship period, you will do so as an out-of-programme research (OOPR) opportunity, and this needs careful planning with your deanery and training programme director.

During your allocated academic time within the ACF, you should aim to accrue generic academic skills such as literature searching, critical analysis, writing abstracts, papers and grant applications. Some candidates will even collect pilot data that will support their grant application and form the foundation of the PhD research project. There is no detailed syllabus directing what skills should be gained and the delivery of the ACF programme remains in the hands of the university to which it is attached. In view of this ACF programmes can be very variable in their quality of formal training, and when applying to one, you should ask the opinions of your colleagues and consultants. In particular you should seek the opinions of the current incumbents. Some trainees may already have a PhD and they are still eligible to apply for ACF posts. These ACFs are expected to restart some research in the allotted time with the aim of applying for intermediate funding and a clinical scientist fellowship, or even CL immediately thereafter. Often the PhD will have been taken years earlier and the ACF academic blocks will allow you to re-introduce yourself to research.

If you fail to obtain funding for a PhD by the end of the 3-year programme, you will simply return to normal clinical training, but can of course continue to apply for a RTF if you wish.

Key points

- Monitor deanery websites and www.nihr.ac.uk for ACF posts
- Is the timing of the academic post appropriate to your training needs?
- Do the academic opportunities available at the institution suit your interests?
- Is the programme well managed?
- Check whether previous post holders achieved a research training fellowship

Where to look for an ACF post

ACF posts provide a fantastic opportunity to learn about and begin to perform research during your clinical training, and they provide previously unavailable structure and stability. The National Institute of Health Research publishes the jobs available in each deanery and each university on its website: http://www.nihr.ac.uk. Look at this website closely and you will see that recruitment is often *prior* to advertisement of clinical posts, but deaneries can advertise at *any time* in the year, and posts can become available at any time for various reasons. This means you will have to be active in pursuing these posts by monitoring the websites closely. This is important because you may be used to the system of once a year applications when everyone is applying for the same thing. You should approach the deanery that interests you to find out exactly when they will advertise and which posts are available as this can vary from year to year. Not all posts are available every year since some deaneries or universities may have ACFs available every second or third year in some specialites.

Academic jobs are available in deaneries across the country and vary at the level at which recruitment occurs. The majority of ACFs are available within speciality training at the level of specialisation (e.g. ST3 in medical specialities or ST1 in paediatrics). For example, you can undertake an ACF post in cardiology or nephrology at ST3 or above. However some are available at core training level, and can be undertaken by CT1, ST1 and ST2 trainees, for example ACF posts in medical education and ACF posts in general medicine. These posts taken earlier in your clinical career may present a real challenge in ensuring you achieve all the core clinical competencies you need and also most likely postgraduate examinations (e.g. MRCP, MRCS), in addition to establishing some research and writing a fellowship application.

Getting the most out of your ACF

It is strongly recommended that upon successfully being awarded an ACF post, that you meet with your ACF co-ordinator and start to meet with potential supervisors. Many previous candidates have waited until their research starts before doing this, meaning their limited allocated research time becomes wasted. Whilst you have a fixed work time to cover research, it is inevitable and necessary to use your spare time (evenings, weekends and annual leave) to ensure your ACF time is fruitful. Whilst this may seem onerous, it's worth considering how long it takes to obtain funding for a PhD (a long time!), and that before the ACF system, it *all* had to be done in your spare time.

Furthermore, you must immediately register with the university library to gain access to journals and the university e-mail system. This will enable you to start researching your ideas before your ACF post officially begins and enable easier communication within the university.

In the first year, you may not have firm ideas of what you want to do long term but by year 2, you should aim to have a research idea developed and have chosen a supervisor. Chapter 8 describes in detail the role of supervisors and the process of applying for a PhD, while Chapter 9 covers funding and research grant applications. Take the advice on board, such that by year 3, you have already applied to a funding body and are awaiting interviews. In years 2 and 3 it would be good to be undertaking active research – collecting data that will help your grant application and even be used as part of your PhD. You should take the opportunity to gain ethics committee approval for your project, and the necessary licenses if animal work is involved.

Planning your time during your ACF is essential to ensure that you are able to balance your academic and clinical training. Your actual plan will be assessed at the Annual Review of Competence Progression (ARCP) and it must be comprehensive and feasible.

Key points – Aims of the ACF

- **Clinical training** – This must be at the same standard of non-academic trainees within each training year. This places the onus on you to squeeze in the same number of cases and procedures required to progress, into a smaller time window
- **Generic academic skills** – There is currently no syllabus available to suggest the skills that are required as an academic trainee. This may change soon. Some deaneries stipulate that trainees take modules or postgraduate qualifications as part of their academic time
- **Application for a clinical research training fellowship** – This is the ultimate aim of an ACF and therefore when planning your ACF you must ensure that you have set time aside for this. There is no absolute rule about the way in which you approach this but the application is a major undertaking and needs time
- **Approach a mentor** – Although many trainees identify a mentor throughout their studies, there are many opportunities to seek out a mentor who is separate from your institution and can give you impartial advice

---

Clinical training

As academic trainees have to achieve the same standards in their clinical training as their clinically trained counterparts, it is advisable to actively seek opportunities to maximise clinical exposure. You should attend clinics and procedural lists that are not on your timetable. Clearly it is an advantage to be good at time management. This is critically important in specialities that require you to have achieved a set numbers of procedures – for example, in cardiology your deanery may stipulate the number of pacemakers to be inserted in a year. You will simply have to work harder because in general, even non-academic trainees have difficulties hitting the target numbers required.

Talk to your local clinical supervisors about the best way to hit your targets. You may need to volunteer to cover other people's shifts.

You must also maintain the same ePortfolio as your non-academic colleagues. Be sure to complete the required number of assessments as this is checked at your ARCP. Failure to do so would normally require you to repeat the year. What is done with the 'academic' component of the year would be at the discretion of your local deanery. It is possible that you may be asked to leave the ACF programme.

Courses and academic skills

Some deaneries and academic supervisors recommend that you undertake modules or postgraduate qualifications. Currently, £1000 per year is available for each academic trainee through their allocated university. This should be used to undertake specialised courses that will further your exposure to research methods and make you a more attractive candidate for a PhD. This funding cannot be used for your actual PhD, so it is worth looking for courses that might help you. For example, if your intended research programme will use ultrasound to assess a physiological principle, then attend a course that teaches and refines your ultrasound technique. Your allocated university will also offer free courses and modules that local PhD students attend; the rules differ but you may be allowed to attend. The deanery will also provide courses open to all ACFs across different disciplines. Furthermore, you should continue to attend the training days for your particular speciality.

If there is a master's programme available in your department, you may be encouraged to undertake it and the fees are sometimes waved. Some trainees undertake a further degree such as a master's and sometimes the timing of these can make it difficult to organise alongside clinical training that is already reduced. When planning these courses, ensure that you reserve enough time during your ACF to take a period of time to plan your grant applications.

If you need to book your own courses and arrange generic teaching then we would recommend the following:

1 **Good Clinical Practice course** – From the EU directive 2001/20/EC, "*Good Clinical Practice is a set of internationally recognised ethical and scientific quality requirements which must be observed for designing, conducting, recording and reporting clinical trials that involve the participation of human subjects.*" Most ethics committees will need to see that you have done a Good Clinical Practice course if you are a principle applicant for ethics approval using human samples. Your university may provide this course; there are national courses and also online courses if you are unable to attend one in person.
2 **Research Governance course** – Research Governance courses overlap with Good Clinical Practice courses, however as well as covering international

standards they will cover the Department of Health Research Governance Framework. The Research Governance Framework for Health and Social Care (RGF) covers core standards including ethics, research and regulatory bodies, accessibility to information, health and safety and financial and intellectual property. If there is a local course at your institution it would be advisable to attend as some institutions have local guidance on research governance.

3 **Statistics course** – It is important to undertake a basic statistics course at the beginning of academic training.

4 **Miscellaneous courses** – There are usually a wide variety of courses available to you as an honorary member of the university. I would take every opportunity to attend ones that you think may be useful, for example presentation skills courses, information technology courses and literature-searching courses. Consider attending those at Royal Colleges that focus on your speciality.

Other important generic skills include writing skills and teaching. Although ACFs outside medical education have no formal role in teaching, you should be actively encouraged to take up roles in teaching within the university and medical school. Your ultimate career path is likely to have a teaching role and therefore developing teaching skills will be invaluable throughout your career.

Application for a clinical research training fellowship

An application for a grant from a respected funding body (a clinical research training fellowship [CRTF]) is the ultimate aim for ACFs. Organisations include the Medical Research Council (MRC) and the Wellcome Trust. This is covered in Chapter 9. You will need to take a period of time (perhaps 3 months) to write an application. These applications are very competitive and trainees in ACF posts have a clear advantage with the amount of time that they can dedicate to an application, so use it wisely. You will be up against other ACF holders and also those who have chosen to apply independently of the ACF system.

Bear in mind that your application may not be successful, so time your applications so that you can have more than one chance to apply during your ACF post. This may sound easy but the applications take several months to process and therefore from submission until decision there may be a lag of 6 or 8 months.

In assessing your application, the funding organisations will consider your potential, the suitability of your supervisors and your project. Choosing your project and supervisor is a major part of your application. In order to get to know potential supervisors, you should get to know other students in their group, attend meetings and perhaps undertake a short project to assess how you work together. This is discussed in more detail in Chapter 8.

Approach a research mentor

A mentor is separate from an educational supervisor or academic supervisor. Some trainees have a self-appointed mentor to guide them through decisions in a confidential and impartial manner.

However, it is occasionally difficult to identify a mentor who is removed from your institution. Therefore there are a number of formal mentoring systems within academic medicine. This includes The Academy of Medical Sciences, which can provide you with a mentor who is separate from your institution and can advise you on the work–life balance and long- and short-term goals within medicine.

Some deaneries also provide a mentoring system. Take these opportunities as there are likely to be frustrations and it can be invaluable to have the advice of someone older and wiser.

Clinical lectureships

Like ACFs, these posts are recruited by the deanery and managed jointly by the NHS trust, university and deanery. The posts are usually for 4 years and comprise a split between academic and clinical time. Again, this varies but can be 50:50. Practically, this is likely to be split as a series of clinical duties spread across the week with the remaining time being academic time. This simply reflects the realities of clinical work but also that you cannot wait for a 6-month gap to get your research off the ground. This emphasises the need for organisation and the need to be strict with your time. It is easy for clinical work to leak into your research time.

The candidates commonly hold an MD or PhD and are looking to pursue an academic career. They should also hold a training number. It is expected that people in these posts apply for further funding and undertake a period of post-doctoral research.

By this stage in your career, you should have most of the generic skills to be a clinician scientist and therefore there is more emphasis on conducting research, developing teaching and supervision skills as well as completing clinical training. This should lead to a series of publications and establish you as researcher in that particular field. You may start to supervise other PhD students, as a co-supervisor initially.

You will still need to finish your clinical training and the ultimate aim is to reach completion of clinical training (Certificate of Completion of Training [CCT] stage). This will allow you to apply for clinician scientist posts at universities and hold an honorary consultant post. From there you will start to run your own research group, whilst still maintaining links with your previous supervisors and mentors.

Key points

National bodies

- **Medical Research Council (www.mrc.ac.uk)** – This is a publicly funded organisation that funds and supports medical research of all types within the UK. It funds physicians and scientists for research
- **National Institute for Health Research (www.nihr.ac.uk)** – This institute was set up to support improvement in infrastructures in medical research within the UK. It offers funding for projects that will directly improve patient care. It also aims to improve the distribution of funding for research by incorporating an open and transparent peer-review system. It provides a list of ACFs and CLs on its website. It also promotes the need for public awareness of medical research. It also runs annual conferences for ACFs and CLs in posts; this allows presentation of data and the opportunity to meet people who are in similar fields
- **Wellcome Trust (www.wellcome.ac.uk)** – The Wellcome Trust funds biomedical, scientific and technological research that aims to improve human health. There are seven subcommittees for different fields of research. Funding is provided to certain universities, who then have local control over which projects and applicants are funded
- **Academy of Medical Sciences (www.acmedsci.ac.uk)** – The Academy of Medical Sciences promotes advances in medical science. It offers support to people interested in following an academic medical career. In doing so it offers a mentor service for ACFs and CLs
- **UK Clinical Research Collaboration (www.ukcrc.org)** – The UK Clinical Research Collaboration is a forum to allow a number of bodies to promote clinical research within the UK and enable the UK to become a world leader in clinical research. These bodies include funding bodies, academic societies, NHS regulatory bodies, patients and industry

Alternative routes into academic medicine

Key points

- Time is always short! Now is the time to *plan* your research
- Be prepared – it can take a long time to get funding
- Start looking at funding bodies as soon as you know you want to do research

Where do I start?

Starting out in research can be a bewildering process. Chapter 2 emphasised that you can start at any stage of your training, and the advantages and disadvantages of the different times. Here we consider how to organise your thoughts and time. The following applies equally to those entering using the

ACF system, but may be more important for those who are entering research from a normal clinical training post with less support and infrastructure.

> **Key point**
> CLAP: **C**onsider, **L**ook, **A**pply, **P**lan.

Consider

Unless you are sure you know exactly what, why and where you want to study, then we recommend considering the following questions. Think long and hard about your answers, these questions will inevitably be asked at an interview with supervisors, funding bodies and your deanery when applying for an OOPR.

1 **Why do you want to do research and what do you hope to get out of it?**
   - Are you interested in further study and/or obtaining a higher degree?
   - Do you see it as a way to improve your CV?
   - Is it a means to an end, i.e. career enhancement?
   - Do you see yourself following an academic career, and if so what does this mean to you? Do you wish to be a full-time academic or do you intend to split your time as a hospital consultant?
   - Are you interested in taking take time out from clinical practice and do you see this as an opportunity to do so whilst maintaining career progression and keeping your options open? Do you see yourself returning to clinical training after this research period?
   - Is this an opportunity to develop an interest, a skill or achieve greater expertise in a particular area?
   - Have you caught the research bug? If so what was your inspiration?
   - Are you attracted to the idea of 'something different' or perhaps are you fulfilling what you believe is an expectation?
   - Are you under the misconception that research may lend itself to a lighter timetable?
   - Do family commitments play a role in your decision?
     Whatever your reasons, ensure you have thought about it as it is likely to influence the type of research you do, the laboratory, team or department, and importantly the supervisor you choose. Furthermore if you are applying for an advertised clinical research position or research funding, you will need to prove your commitment to research and justify your reasons for taking time out of clinical training. You will need to ensure your CV reflects your commitment to research (see Chapter 5) and that you can 'tick' as many 'boxes' as you can on both the essential and desired criterion for any research post you wish take.
2 **Why did you not decide to apply for an ACF post if you want to do research?** This is a deliberately provocative question and only relevant since

the introduction of ACFs. It is however something you may need to justify. There are a number of reasons, practical and personal. For example, there are only a limited number of ACFs and a candidate may not want to define their path early in their career. You may have developed your interest later during your training having been inspired by another project. It may be borne out of a desire to specialise in a particular area. Equally, it is possible that you simply did not have enough exposure to research and academia when you were applying for training posts and therefore you opted not to apply for an ACF. There may of course not have been any ACFs in your speciality or geographic region. Equally, you may have applied for an ACF but were not successful. If this is the case it does demonstrate a commitment to research and therefore you could use it to your advantage when applying for a research post.

Not having an ACF should not put you off applying for an OOPR/E and/or taking a detour down the 'academic route'. An individual's interest can be sparked at any stage in their career. Someone who has made an active, informed and impassioned decision to apply for a research fellowship in a particular area of interest should be encouraged and will find support.

3 **What type of research are you interested in?** There are many options and a variety of opportunities available for an OOPE. This is your chance to do something unique and should be a personal choice. Do not be put off by taking an unconventional path if it suits you or choosing something very different to your peers.

- **Laboratory/clinical based or a bit of both?** Do you see yourself in the laboratory working closely with scientists at the cutting edge of their field developing a proof of concept or new scientific discovery? For example you could study the flow of calcium into myocardial cells to understand the role of calcium receptors in heart failure. Alternatively you may want to conduct a scientific study using patients as the study subjects, scanning heart failure patients to see if you could find a variable that explains why some respond to certain drugs and not others. Clearly both are research into heart failure, but at very different ends of the spectrum. If one makes you recoil in horror, then that kind of research is not for you!

Remember that most research conducted by doctors is 'clinical' and will always involve some contact with patients, even if you are in a laboratory every day studying cells. You may need to collect human tissue during surgery or in clinic. Alternatively, your research programme may require you to run a clinic or perform a diagnostic/therapeutic list which could have the added advantage of enhancing your skills. Bear in mind that if you are aiming for a full time academic career and ultimately a professional post, then Basic Science Research may be the most appropriate.

- **Running/coordinating clinical trials?** Do you see yourself recruiting patients into a study of different chemotherapy agents – identifying those who may benefit, recruiting and consenting them, then following them up over time and collecting data on them? This is unlikely to lead to a PhD but remains an important and valuable clinical research activity.

- **Working abroad?** Medicine continues to provide many opportunities to go abroad. You can go to do research or a clinical fellowship to learn a new skill, or just take part of your normal training programme abroad. In general, this takes a great deal of organisation and you will need determination and the support of your training directors as well as funding. Get planning early (see Chapter 12).
- **Diplomas/MSc** Perhaps you want to develop an interest but would rather not commit to a MD/PhD. An option may be a specialist Msc. An increasingly popular alternative, and one which is regarded highly in a consultant interview, is a Diploma in Medical Education. Something which may become more relevant, particularly in light of recent changes in the structure of the NHS, is an MBA (Masters of Business Administration). Diplomas and Msc courses are covered in Chapter 7.

4 **What field are you interested in studying?** Although not always the case, remember your OOPE/R is likely to influence and define your future career. The later in your training that you take it, the greater the clinical link. For example, Cardiologists interested in the subspeciality of electrophysiology may undertake a PhD in a particular arrhythmia treatment. This would then support them when applying for subspeciality training and consultant posts in electrophysiology. However if you take an OOPR early, your research area can be totally unrelated to what you 'grow up' to be. Whilst the subject area may not apply, the transferable skills will be invaluable to your future career.

5 **When should you take your OOPE/R – early or late in your specialist training?** This decision may depend on why you are considering research. If you are interested in a career in academia and aim to apply for an academic position post CCT then you may want to consider research later in your training (during higher training rather than in the foundation years or core training). This would have the advantage that you are in the right position to apply for a post-doctorate research training grant in order to continue your academic career without having to return to years of clinical training. Bear in mind that unless there are exceptional circumstances it is unlikely you will be allowed to take an OOPE period in your last year of clinical training.

Alternatively, you may want to define your specialist interest early in your career and having a higher degree, publications and/or area of particular expertise will allow you to stand out from your colleagues, provide the skills to continue research, set up your own projects, publish throughout clinical training and/or develop a niche.

If you are not interested in pursuing an academic career post CCT, you may want to consider your OOPE early in your training. You may find yourself clinically de-skilled after taking time out of specialist registrar (SpR) training if you do not continue 'on-calls'/specialist clinics/lists/training and maintain skills during your research period.

> **Key points – Realistic timelines**
>
> | | |
> |---|---|
> | Looking for a supervisor/lab/research project: | 1 year |
> | Getting to know lab, research, techniques and writing a grant application: | 6 months |
> | From application to interview: | 4–6 months |
> | From award of grant to leaving: | 3–6 months |
>
> (it can however be up to 12 months as many deaneries only allow you to leave a training post once a year)

Look

Spend time looking around and network with colleagues, predecessors in research and academic mentors.

1 **Speak to your senior colleagues** – This is time well spent and you will gain a wealth of advice. Ask their opinion regarding:
    - What and where they carried out their research
    - Did they enjoy it; was it productive, were they supported?
    - Could they recommend a supervisor/team?
    - Are their labs/supervisors looking for potential PhD/MD candidates?
    - Are they about to advertise a research post?
2 **Visit labs, institutes, teaching hospitals** – Explore the options available for research, develop contacts, express your interest and gain advice. Remain motivated.
3 **Attend speciality training days, forums, symposiums, conferences** – These are useful to find out what research is current and on the horizon. Discover what sparks your interest. Speak to the scientists/specialists after their presentation and show your interest. Networking is essential in academia.
4 **Make appointments to see supervisors** – Approach supervisors directly. Find out what is available and whether there are new projects you could get involved in or take on. Ensure you have read their latest publications and are aware of their current research. Be enthusiastic, determined and show commitment. Remember you will be spending 2–3 years with your supervisor. It is important that you are happy in your new environment, it suits your disposition and you get on with the boss and team. As such it is important to spend time in the lab/department and chat with the previous Fellows prior to making your final decision. A happy lab is essential for your sanity and cannot be underestimated. Supervisors are covered in detail in Chapter 8.

5 **Look out for advertised positions** – If a lab receives a project/programme grant then they may advertise for a research fellow to carry out the work. Many research posts are advertised locally in the university careers pages so keep an eye out. Consult especially:
   - *British Medical Journal*
   - Speciality coordinator in the deanery, who may forward advertised positions
   - University career pages.

Remember that applying to an advertised post will require you to pay attention to your CV and the application form. Practice your interview skills. Visit the department before your interview and talk to the supervisor, just as you would if you were formulating your own research project. Some funded posts last only a short time (such as year), but will enable you to get pilot data for other grant applications. Other programmes are available with 'soft money', which comes out the department's coffers if they particularly like you. In this case, you should also take the opportunity to seek alternative funding to ensure you have sufficient funds available to cover your salary and potential laboratory and research costs.

Apply

Historically trainees could start a project without funding in place. This is not the case anymore. For an OOPE to be accepted by the deanery you have to provide confirmation that funding is in place before you leave your clinical training post ideally for the whole duration of the research. Funding is covered in detail in Chapter 9 but briefly:

1 **You can apply for a funded position or project** – A lab may have money from a programme grant that they can spend on a research trainee, or a supervisor may have written a grant application for a particular project and already have funding for a clinician to carry out the project. These positions will be advertised. Obviously if you have shown interest previously that will work to your advantage. Often these positions are only for 2 years but if the trainee wishes to extend the project to a PhD they can apply for a further year's funding. Many charitable organisations offer funding for 1 year.

2 **Apply for your own funding** – Some consider this route has more academic kudos than a pre-funded project, because you have worked to obtain the funding and it is specifically allocated to you. A number of organisations can provide funding through a competitive process:
   - Charitable organisations – organisations with a specialist interest or university charities (e.g. Cancer UK, British Heart Foundation, Kidney Research UK, Action Research).
   - National Institute for Health Research – the central Government-backed funding body particularly funds projects that are generally under-represented by other funding bodies.

- Large funding bodies – MRC and Wellcome Trust. The application process is identical regardless of whether you have an ACF or are taking an independent route.
- Pharmaceutical companies – this is increasingly difficult unless the funding has already been won by the research group.

Funding applications will require writing a 'grant application', which is covered in detail in Chapter 9. This takes time and concerted effort and will not be easy. Without being in an ACF post, this will all have to be done in your own time (weekends, evenings, annual leave). You will need to take time off work to meet with supervisors. It helps to have a sympathetic clinical boss who may have gone through the same process.

If your application is unsuccessful, try again! It is not uncommon that a candidate is unsuccessful the first time round. Try to make yourself more competitive for the next round.

Key points

If your application is unsuccessful:
- **Debrief** – ask for feedback after an interview
- **Improve your CV** – write up that abstract/paper you never got around to. Get involved in a clinical trial (you will gain experience and demonstrate your interest and commitment to research). Do a Good Clinical Practice course (a requirement for anyone involved in a clinical research project). Show that you understand what is involved in clinical research and the standards you must meet. Attend meetings and forums on the subject you are interested in researching
- **Re-write your grant application** – perhaps your project needs re-vamping or needs to be more focussed. Discuss this with your supervisor and take advice. Again, you may get some useful feedback after the interview. Embrace constructive criticism
- **Arrange a practice interview**
- **Apply to a different funding body or research department**
- **Above all do not lose heart, prove your determination and persevere**

Plan

Once you have chosen a supervisor and research team you will need to plan your OOP time carefully:

1 Keep your deanery informed and updated. In the first instance, let them know you are looking for research and take advice as to when you will be allowed out of the programme. Most deaneries will only allow trainees out on a clinical changeover date (e.g. February, April, August or October) so as not to leave a hospital uncovered without a specialist registrar. There are exceptions, but this will need to be negotiated with the training programme director. They are likely to be more accommodating and sympathetic if they

have had ample notice. Minimum notice is 3 months but expect to have to give 6.

2 Inform the deanery and your training programme director when you are applying for either a funded research post or training fellowship (MRC/Wellcome) and/or have an interview. Once you have been awarded the post or funding there may be a deadline as to when the position/award must be taken up and the deanery can refuse to let you 'out of programme' if you have not given sufficient notice, and if your clinical training is not progressing satisfactorily.

3 Find out the contractual notice that is required for you to resign from your position at your hospital trust. Usually this is 3 months.

Key points

- An ACF is not essential, but without one the process will consume more of your personal time and require more effort, and you may not have a chance to acquire some research experience or pilot data
- The application process is lengthy
- Show dedication and persevere
- Keep your deanery informed and up to date with your plans

Case studies

Dr Jonathan Coombs

A Gastroenterology SpR, Dr Coombs started looking for research at the end of his ST3 year. He attended educational meetings, speciality forums and an international conference in order to see what current research was being carried out and to meet potential supervisors. He became involved in a multi-centre trial in his ST4 year to gain clinical research experience and attended a Good Clinical Practice course to understand the standards set for clinical research practitioners. He applied for a funded clinical research fellow position, which was advertised though the deanery. He was shortlisted for an interview, which included a presentation. He managed to take some annual leave to prepare by swapping on-calls and offering to cover other colleagues' endoscopy lists and clinics. He dedicated his spare time towards the interview and met supervisors involved in the research project. Unfortunately Dr Coombs was not successful. However feedback from the interview was positive and encouraged him to keep looking for a research post. He was recommended 1 year later to a supervisor who was looking for a new research fellow to run his clinical trial. Together they wrote a grant application to the National Institute for Health Research (NIHR) and acquired funding for 2 years. Dr Coombs started his research post in his ST6 year and whilst in post applied for a further year's funding and achieved a PhD. He later returned to clinical training and continued to be involved in clinical trials with his supervisor.

Dr Seema Kumar

A 3rd year respiratory SpR (ST5) approached a supervisor and arranged a meeting following an interesting lecture at a training day. Dr Kumar read around the subject and relevant papers published by the lab and had an informal chat with the research team before the meeting. The supervisor was impressed by Dr Kumar's enthusiasm and suggested a possible research project. Together they developed this idea over the following 8 months and put together a grant application, which they sent to the large funding bodies. Dr Kumar attended the lab on a regular basis to get to grips with the techniques she would be using and understand the hurdles she would face. She got shortlisted by the Wellcome Trust 5 months later. She had 2 weeks' notice for the interview and had taken annual leave in order to prepare. She spent every day in the lab and her supervisor organised a mock interview. She was awarded a research training fellowship for 3 years following a successful interview, which could be taken up immediately. As she was in a clinical training post and a replacement could not be found she was not able to take up the research position until October of that year. She returned to her final year of clinical training after completing her PhD.

Ms Natalie Smith

Ms Smith is a Colorectal Surgeon at the end of her 3rd year of higher speciality training, Ms Smith was interested in learning a new technique abroad. She contacted a senior colleague who had been on a similar secondment and had connections in Australia. She arranged the attachment via email and had a telephone interview for a clinical fellow position. She put together a proposal that was accepted by her deanery, who agreed the OOPE she had organised was an appropriate training opportunity. She was able to take 1 year out of programme at the end of her fourth year. Whilst in Australia she ran a clinical trial in this new technique she had set up with her Australian supervisor before she left. Her supervisor organised both the ethics approval and funding for the trial. She was paid as a clinical fellow and joined the on-call rota to supplement her pay. She wrote up the trial and published it on her return to England, where she continued to develop the technique and her new area of expertise.

Dr Stephen Morris

Dr Morris had been on an academic foundation programme and had become enthused by the renal project he had undertaken. He had completed core medical training, passing his MRCP exams at the first sitting and spent his spare time on further work with the renal laboratory. He applied for a renal ACF advertised during his CT2 year, which he gained, and started out in a clinical renal post. He spent the first 3-month academic block in two different research groups at the university learning some techniques, deciding what sort of work he liked and talking with the various potential supervisors, before settling on a study of a new animal model and its underlying pathogenesis and investigating a novel therapeutic intervention. In his second 3-month academic block he established some preliminary data, applied for an animal licence and wrote an application with his supervisor for an MRC training fellowship, which he won. He started his OOPR after his ST4 year ended. His research was very successful and he remained enthused, then he applied for a CL starting immediately after his CRTF. He won the CL post but could not start for 6 months, so returned to a clinical post initially. His research periods were then taken as 6-month blocks although he remained on call for 1 in 4 weekends during the research time. He planned to continue this for 3 years and then apply for a Clinician Scientist award or if advertised a 'new blood' senior lectureship.

4

Research in surgical training

Joseph Shalhoub

Statistics suggest that surgical specialities have differing views on academic careers when compared to other medical specialities. Whilst historically a period of research was expected of trainees in order to secure senior posts, the current role of research in surgical training remains unclear and there are varying opinions. The Society for Academic and Research Surgery (SARS), the various deaneries and the surgical Royal Colleges have all provided their own approach to disseminate information about the value of research in surgical training. This chapter hopes to share some of the information accrued from these sources, as well as personal experiences of undertaking research in surgery.

Significant statistical difference

Whilst there has been a modest reduction in the number of clinical academics in the UK overall, the most marked reduction has been in surgery. The number of surgical trainees with academic numbers has halved since 2000. Furthermore, only 9% of clinical academics are surgeons, compared to 37% who are physicians. At present less than 2% of the UK's medical research funding is awarded to surgery-based research projects. The Royal College of Surgeons of England has recognised this and developed a new syllabus as 'a desperate need to redress this balance'.

Surgical training curriculum

The Intercollegiate Surgical Curriculum Programme (ISCP) is the surgical training syllabus and features a research curriculum at both core (generally CT1–CT2) and speciality (generally ST3–ST8) training levels. The research areas are also formally assessed in the viva component of the Intercollegiate FRCS 'exit examination'; this demands an understanding of the literature and interpretation of publications for evidence-based practice. Furthermore, it is clear that the transferable skills acquired through undertaking research can contribute to the making of a good surgeon.

Clearly some surgeons will wish to be clinician scientists, attain a PhD on the way to a senior lecturer position and ultimately professorial position. For many though conducting research as a trainee will help to 'tick boxes' and complete sections of their training portfolio, and will also provide time management, organisation and perseveration skills. Manual dexterity can also be maintained and developed (depending on the research project undertaken). Some aspects of research, including animal models, are technically demanding. For example, developing rodent models of hydronephrosis may require ligating tiny ureters. Many core surgical skills can be developed including dissection, knot tying, suturing and performing anastomoses on a small scale and perhaps under an operating microscope with fine microsurgical instruments.

Surgical pathways and research opportunities

Research can be pursued in a trainee's own time, alongside clinical posts, or during part-time or full-time degree courses (see Chapter 7), or as part of an ACF (see Chapter 3) programme. Clearly the amount that can be achieved working on a project while holding down a full-time clinical post is limited and would not amount to pursuing an academic career in its own right, although will of course be useful in a number of ways. The numbers of students undertaking MB-PhD programmes are small and thus, in reality your first chance for research will be during an intercalated BSc or equivalent. To truly advance your career in surgery, you should start demonstrating a research interest early, during an intercalated degree or in your foundation years.

Foundation doctors on an 'academic programme' have a fantastic opportunity to spend 3–4 months in research, and there are such opportunities specifically offering surgical research around the UK. Dedicated surgical programmes are not widespread so hunt them out. If you are seriously interested in a career in surgery then your productivity during this time is critical, and you must be able to show what you achieved. Applying for training in surgical programmes is incredibly competitive and you will be expected to have produced publications, pilot data or at least a significant audit in this time. An ACF post should give you a significant advantage although there have been examples in the past, when motivated non-academic foundation doctors have produced more research output (having done this in their own time) than academic foundation doctors (who have their 4-month 'academic block', and their spare time for the remaining 20 months). Don't forget that all the necessary clinical competencies need to be attained in this shorter time for those in academic training, serving to highlight the 'shift' from time-determined to competency-based progression in clinical training. Focus on surgical research and seek out a surgical academic clinician to mentor you during your F2 programme (whether academic or not).

Pitfalls

- Don't sit on your laurels! An academic post on your CV alone will not bring you any kudos! You have to do the work and produce research and/or publications

---

In the recent past, it was common for senior house officers (SHOs) seeking a surgical training programme (SpR) to undertake a higher degree programme before applying. This is less common now and F2 doctors can apply directly to a core surgical training programme (CT1) without doing this. You should also consider the ACF posts, and some are on offer in surgery. As described in Chapter 3, ACF posts have protected time and support to produce fellowship applications and allow you to obtain funding for a higher degree. This represents a fantastic opportunity and you should look at the NIHR and deanery websites for details of surgical programmes around the UK. It should be remembered that those who do not 'get on' in research can always revert back to a standard clinical training post. Again, it must be emphasised that surgical competencies will still have to be obtained but in a shortened time frame. You will have to be responsible for your own clinical training, seeking out opportunities and maximising them.

Research degrees

In the past it was common for surgical trainees to undertake an MD (2 years, full time). This is changing, and for many a 1-year master's is more applicable for your career aims (see Chapter 7). For a formal career in academic surgery though a research degree is important if not essential, and undertaking a PhD (3 years, full time) has become increasingly popular. In some geographical areas, a PhD or MD has become almost essential to gain a consultant post in major (teaching) hospitals.

When to do formal research

Most surgical consultants would be happy to support the undertaking of informal research, in some form, from an early stage. The debate over 'early' research (during or before core surgical training) versus late (close to consultant appointment) remains unresolved and will depend on individual circumstances and real career aims. In a similar manner to medical specialities, the later you do your research, the more integrated it may be to your long-term clinical aims. For example, if you have decided to become a colorectal surgeon you could perform a focused PhD on the use of molecular dyes during surgery to distinguish malignant from normal tissue, or an MD on a specific laparoscopic technique. However undertaking a PhD after core surgical training in a cancer laboratory on the biology of telomeres (i.e. very basic research), could be a prelude to an academic career in any surgical speciality. In reality most surgical academics tend to undertake research rather directly linked to their practice. Early research will help you obtain a surgical training post, but is much less likely to be related to your long-term career. A surgery-based project will demonstrate 'commitment' to a surgical career. It will help build a network of contacts and collaborations that prove invaluable when applying for training posts. Furthermore, as you begin to supervise other research projects, this will elevate your own research as well as your skill set. You are also more likely to achieve excellence in research if you start early!

New directions in surgical training

Further changes to the surgical curriculum may also support the direct integration of research into surgical training. The London School of Surgery is considering the introduction of a third core training year (CT3) to allow further refinement of surgical skills in your chosen speciality while also completing the core modules of three master's degrees (MSc in Surgical Science, an MEd in Medical Education, and an MA in Medical Ethics and Law). This would provide the trainees with a flavour of the different 'types' of academia and research, and a springboard to develop an interest in these areas further. Once these trainees move into a speciality training post from CT3, they will go on to complete one of these master's degrees. Some trainees can then choose to obtain funding for a full-time PhD. This model is still developing and it is unclear whether or not it will be adopted in its entirety. It does, however demonstrate that a higher degree is not necessary for the attainment of a core or higher surgical training post.

Types of research

Surgical research can be clinical or more laboratory based, basic or applied, or can focus on clinical trials, imaging, technologies or much more. Surgical specialities lend themselves to translational research, which is currently in vogue. There is also the opportunity for 'hybrid' research, combining basic science such as molecular and cellular biology together with clinical research. Non-scientific research remains an option for surgical trainees. Surgeons have conducted research into educational, management and leadership techniques. This is expanding and encouraged in the hope that the clinical teachers and managers of the future may have their credentials in these areas formalised. For example, the surgeon Professor Lord Darzi, during his time as Under-Secretary of State for Health, established the Darzi Fellowship programme. Darzi Fellows "participate in a bespoke leadership development programme that aims to support the organisational and leadership skills necessary for their future roles as consultants and clinical leaders".

There is a question, of a 'chicken and egg' nature, around whether to base your research around clinical aspirations, or your clinical focus around research interests. There are a spectrum of answers to this with some individuals at one extreme targeting a particular speciality and driving both their clinical and academic pursuits towards this with narrow focus, overcoming often considerable competition and challenges to achieve the optimum path to their desired and pre-defined career. On the other end are those who follow opportunities as they present and take a 'path of least resistance'. Most people select their research and career paths somewhere in between these two extremes, with a number of trainees selecting rotations that allow them to explore potential specialties of interest, then build their research around 'hot topics' in this speciality, or fields within that speciality where local expertise and facilities exist. Trainees also build on their prior experience, for example taking forward BSc projects, continuing the work they started having often selected the speciality or area of medicine by selecting the BSc programme in the first place.

Pitfalls in surgical research

- Ethics approval is time consuming and can delay you considerably
- Ensure you complete a Good Clinical Practice course
- Animal work will need Home Office training and a license
- Funding is essential and you will need to apply early

Supervisors and mentors in surgical research

The importance of mentorship and good academic supervision in surgical research cannot be overstated. A surgical academic mentor should be a role model, and can be separate from a clinical and academic supervisor. The mentor can help provide impartial advice over prolonged periods of time, understand how research and training can combine and listen to you, helping you to overcome hurdles. Choosing your supervisor is of course as important in surgery as in other disciplines (see Chapters 8 and 13). Consider carefully their research group and facilities, track record including successful research students, grants, ongoing projects, recent publications (including the impact factors of the journals published in) and whether they have time to supervise you properly. Visiting the supervisor and their unit before committing yourself means that there should be no surprises when arriving on the first day of your research appointment.

> **Key points**
> - Seek out your deanery and training programme director's advice on research in surgery
> - Attend the London Deanery School of Surgery Academic Careers day (or local deanery day if one exists)

Disadvantages of research in surgery

In the early years of an academic pathway, some trainees may be deterred by 'unbanded' academic blocks in their training, where they are often paid less than their non-academic colleagues as they do not participate in the on-call rota. This should not discourage you and is easier to bear in reality earlier than later in a career! You also have to attain your clinical competencies in less time, for example foundation programme competencies in 20 months as compared with 24 months as 4 months are spent on an academic attachment. Surgery is, arguably more than other areas of medicine, an experience-dependent, technically demanding craft speciality, and research comes at the cost of clinical development. It is said that surgical trainees can 'deskill' whilst in research jobs. Make full use of simulation and other tools to enhance the time available to you. Some feel that the possible compromise of clinical training may be attenuated by retaining some clinical commitments during research. On-call periods or outpatient clinics will keep the clinical part of the brain active, offer opportunities for operative experience, skills maintenance and acquisition, and supplement your income. Furthermore, if your research is clinical this will facilitate patient enrolment into studies. Conversely, clinical commitments can place time pressures on research. Make sure you balance these carefully and do not spread yourself too thinly.

During more senior years, there is a degree of job vulnerability in academia. There is a pressure from the academic institution (often a university) to publish papers in journals with a high-impact factor and bring in research funding. During economically labile periods, there have been some high-profile redundancies of university non-clinical and clinical academics. Clinically there is pressure on waiting lists, outpatient clinics and clinical governance issues, and living with both masters can be difficult, possibly more so in surgery than medicine. Finally, there are fewer posts available for academic surgery at senior levels and less research funding available, putting further strains on advancing in academia as a surgeon. You will have less time as a consultant surgeon for private practice.

> **Key points**
>
> The following are supportive organisations with information on research during surgical training:
>
> - Society for Academic and Research Surgery (SARS) – www.surgicalresearch.org.uk
> - Association of Surgeons in Training (ASiT, who have an academic surgical representative from SARS on their Council) – www.asit.org
> - Association of Surgeons of Great Britain and Ireland – www.asgbi.org
> - Royal College of Surgeons of England – www.rcseng.ac.uk
> - Royal College of Surgeons of Edinburgh – www.rcsed.ac.uk
> - Royal College of Physicians and Surgeons of Glasgow – www.rcpsg.ac.uk
> - Royal College of Physicians in Ireland – www.rcsi.ie
> - ISCP – www.iscp.ac.uk
> - Royal Society of Medicine – www.rsm.ac.uk
> - National Institute for Health Research Trainees' Coordinating Centre (regarding the academic training pathway) – www.nihrtcc.nhs.uk

Conclusions

Formal research during surgical training is now embedded to some extent within the current surgical curriculum, and is supported by surgical and trainee organisations, as well as trainees themselves. This is clearly important in ensuring surgeons have a basic understanding and knowledge of research, but does not make up for encouraging more surgeons to undertake periods of full-time research aiming for academic surgical careers. There is considerable flexibility as regards the timing, discipline and level of research during surgical training. When making decisions regarding research surgical trainees need to consider their career aspirations, interests, the opportunities, and potential supervisors, mentors, academic units and funding streams.

Further reading

Brass LF, Akabas MH, Burnley LD, Engman DM, Wiley CA, Andersen OS. Are MD-PhD programs meeting their goals? An analysis of career choices made by graduates of 24 MD-PhD programs. *Acad Med* 85(4):692–701

Darzi Fellowship. http://www.london.nhs.uk/what-we-do/developing-nhs-staff/leading-for-health/darzi-fellowship

Frank JR, Langer B. Collaboration, communication, management, and advocacy: teaching surgeons new skills through the CanMEDS Project. *World J Surg* 2003;27(8):972–8; discussion 978

Gordon C, Salmon M. Postgraduate degrees for rheumatology trainees: an options appraisal of MD, PhD and MSc degrees. On behalf of the BSR

Research and Training Committee. *Rheumatology (Oxford)* 1999;38(12): 1290–3

Intercollegiate Surgical Curriculum Programme. www.iscp.ac.uk, 2010

Margerison CM, H. *Clinical Academic Staffing Levels in* UK *Medical and Dental Schools.* Medical Schools Council (previously The Council of Heads of Medical Schools) and the Council of Heads and Deans of Dental Schools, 2007

Research Department TRCoSoE. Surgical Research Report 2010–2011. *Investing in Research to Improve Patient Welfare,* 2009

The Royal College of Physicians and Surgeons of Canada. *The CanMEDS 2005 Physician Competency Framework,* 2005

Shalhoub J, Sikkel MB. The attributes of a good medical trainee: how to build your portfolio. *Br J Hosp Med (Lond)* 2009;70(6):M92–5

Society for Academic and Research Surgery (SARS). The Place of Research and Other Educational Experience in UK Surgical Training: Guidance for Surgical Trainees, in Issues in Professional Practice, 2010

5

Academic curriculum vitae

Sukhjinder S Nijjer
Jasdeep K Gill
Jeremy B Levy
Philip J Smith

An academic curriculum vitae (CV) plays an essential role when applying for a higher degree and later to secure clinical lectureship posts and other permanent academic positions. A potential supervisor will certainly ask for your CV to ascertain your past achievements before considering you for a project. You will need to attach your CV to a grant or fellowship application form for funding or when seeking an already funded research post. Therefore your CV is your first opportunity to promote and sell yourself. It must demonstrate your past experience, present academic achievements and more importantly your academic *potential*.

You must remember that your CV is not a static document. As your experiences and achievements grow, so too should your CV. Take a moment to look at your CV, consider how it could be modified and improved to get you *that* post, project or funding. This chapter should prompt you to identify gaps on your CV that are commonly assessed during your career in academic medicine.

■ Structuring your academic CV

The recommended length and format for an academic CV will vary. Often two pages are described as the standard length for a CV at a more junior stage in a career, but there is no 'right' length for an academic CV, and all will depend on where you are in your career, what you are using it for and what you need to demonstrate. There are three distinct styles of academic CV that may be needed in different scenarios. The shorter variants can be attached to certain grant applications to emphasise your background and potential to complete the project proposed, but read any instructions carefully.

1 1-page CVs – Focus on recent grants, papers and prizes with a very brief career summary.
2 2-page CVs – Include the above but also educational achievements and a personal statement.
3 Full CVs – Include everything!

Provided you are not including irrelevant details or have been asked to submit only a 1-page CV, then you should not be concerned if your CV extends onto more than 2 pages. Make sure you submit what is asked of you.

You should tailor your CV for the specific post or purpose. This often involves rearranging the order of information presented on the page, but sometimes it can require a rewrite of particular sections to highlight skills that are specifically relevant to your application. For example, you may have previously used an example of audit to demonstrate your teamwork skills, but now need to modify that example to demonstrate your data collection, statistical and analytical skills. Remember, you must always highlight *your* role and involvement in a project if it involves a team, but you must never lie or exaggerate your involvement.

Beware!
- Never lie or fabricate anything on your CV
- Don't be tempted to use a fancy font or busy layout
- Don't leave the preparation of your CV until the last minute
- Read and re-read your CV before submitting; spelling mistakes and other errors can easily creep in and do not impress

The format of your CV should allow it to be easily read. Its overall design should be individual to you but conservative. Your word-processor may have a wide range of templates for CVs, which can sometimes be mind-boggling and should not generally be used! You should avoid having a busy layout, which may appear to be eye-catching but could distract the reader from your achievements and the actual content of your CV, and will annoy some readers. You must avoid the temptation to use a creative or fancy font that may be difficult for others to read. Common fonts used are Times New Roman or Arial. You should use one font and make use of different font size and bold, underline or italic features to highlight headings or specific information.

Key points
- Use **bold** and *italics* sparsely and appropriately: for example, to draw the readers eye to your contribution on a publication, i.e. Smith AP, **Montgomery LS**, Swan P, Singh A. The change in QTC dispersion affects the likelihood of drug-induced Torsardes de Pointes. *J Cardiol* 2010;15:192–6

- Avoid flashy fonts or overly graphical designs. Use a straightforward 'plain'-looking CV that emphasises your academic achievements and potential, rather than an eye-catching but confusing one!

Be cautious in using flamboyant designs and colours. Light greys and black bold reproduces well in laser-printed copies of your CV. Knowing how to use 'tabs' and aligning all the sections is essential: not only will the document be much easier on the eye but it demonstrates your IT prowess. Trainees are often unsure about whether or not to include their photograph as part of their academic CV. This is really a matter of personal choice unless explicitly requested, usually for security reasons of confirming identity. Generally your aim should be to spoon-feed the reader and demonstrate to them that you meet their criteria using your CV. Keep it simple and succinct.

Full CV

The areas to include in a full CV are listed below. You should submit your full CV, unless otherwise specified. The sequence of your CV is important to consider. Your CV should read as a story and highlight chronology of events. Having a clear structure to your CV will help the reader follow the sequence of events.

Your 'full CV' you should include:

1 Front cover (not crucial).
2 Contents page (not crucial especially at an early stage of a career).
3 Personal details.
4 Academic background.
5 Research history.
6 Courses attended.
7 Audit.
8 Teaching.
9 Career summary.

Think carefully about your experiences and achievements. There should be something positive you can write in each section. For example, if you have no publications yet, you could include those in preparation or submitted that are awaiting decision, but you must ensure these are clearly marked as such. The first page of your CV should be *high impact* if possible and therefore include prizes, grants and major publications in peer-reviewed journals. If you have to prepare a short CV, then these must be on the first page for impact. This will produce a 'halo effect', where all your further achievements are seen in a positive light.

Front page

The front page should be simple, with your name and qualifications. Use a large font size, the current date and ensure the CV is up to date (see Example 5.1). You may wish to put 'In application for the post of…' to demonstrate that you are organised and have tailored your CV for that particular post (but check this for each submission!) Using last year's CV or having the wrong job title on the front cover will look incredibly poor. Remember that doing research requires organisation and using a systematic approach. Don't fall down on the front page!

Example 5.1

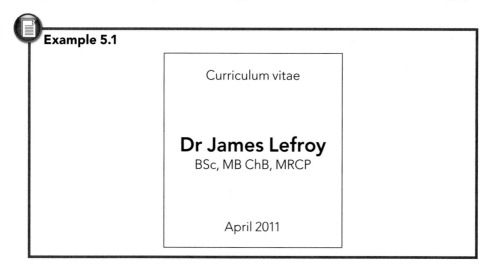

Curriculum vitae

Dr James Lefroy
BSc, MB ChB, MRCP

April 2011

Contents page

Whilst short CVs do not need a contents page, they can be useful in a longer full CV. Create them in a table or use tabs to ensure correct alignment. Some word processors can automate this provided you have been consistent with fonts and styles for headings. Ensure it is up to date when you change your CV. Do not forget to number your pages so that the reader can directly turn to a specific page they may be interested in.

Personal details

This can be formatted in a number of ways: a separate page is reasonable in a long CV, or in shorter CVs a boxed section in the top left or right corner may help so that more high-impact information can fit onto the first page.

The following are all self-explanatory:

* Name – If you are more known by another name give that also.
* Date of birth.
* Nationality.
* GMC number.
* NTN – State your national training number, if you have one, and give the deanery.
* Address – Give your postal address.
* Telephone – Give both your mobile and landline if possible.
* E-mail – A permanent e-mail that is accessible on the go (e.g. via a smartphone). Remember that not all trusts allow you to access accounts such as 'hotmail' or 'yahoo'.

Academic background

Education and qualifications

As you become more senior you supersede the importance of previous educational achievements. List your secondary school and universities(s) in chronological order with your completed degrees. School and school qualifications obviously become irrelevant as your progress beyond the earliest stages of clinical training, so drop them. Include your intercalated BSc degree if you have one, or other undergraduate qualifications. Give the degree class (1st, 2:1, 2:2, 3rd) and report honours if you received it for your medical degree. Give your completed college exams (MRCP, MRCS etc.).

Postgraduate diplomas are excellent at showing your commitment to your speciality of choice and your ability to focus your mind outside of the university environment! It takes special effort to perform these when you're working full time in clinical work (see Example 5.2).

Example 5.2

* **Example with date first (left)**

2007	MRCP (UK)	Royal College of Physicians, London
2006	DTM&H	Diploma of Tropical Medicine & Hygiene, University of London
2000–2001	BSc (Hons)	1st Class (intercalated, Pharmacology)
1998–2004	MBBS (Hons)	University of Newcastle Medical School
1990–1997	GCSEs/A-Levels	St Andrew's Grammar School, Letchworth

- **Example with date last (right)**

MRCP (UK)	Royal College of Physicians, London	2007
DTM&H	Diploma of Tropical Medicine & Hygiene	2006
BSc (Hons)	1st Class (intercalated, Pharmacology)	2000–2001
MBBS (Hons)	University of Newcastle Medical School	1998–2004
GCSEs/A-Levels	St Andrew's Grammar School, Letchworth	1990–1997

You should consider the order and where you put information on the page. Bearing in mind that in English we read from left to right, the reader's eye will be naturally drawn to the left side of the page first. So you should aim to put the most important information or high-impact words on the left side of the page. The hierarchy of information should start with your first achievements, where and then when. Some people advocate putting the date at the right-hand side of the page because it is considered the least important piece of information. Whereas others prefer dates down the left. This is completely up to you!

Prizes

All prizes are a sign of excellence and should be emphasised (Example 5.3). Some may need explanation if the title is eponymous to explain why it was awarded. List all information in reverse-chronological order. In shorter CVs where space is a commodity, focus on those prizes relevant for your chosen speciality.

Example 5.3

- 2008   Anaesthesia Essay Prize – *Runner-up*
         Royal Society of Medicine, Anaesthesia
- 2004   Dermatology Prize
         Awarded for best performance in Dermatology
- 2002   Stanley Blakemore Prize
         Awarded for highest exam mark in Pathology

If you have no prizes, then now is the time to apply for some! The Royal Colleges, Royal Society of Medicine and a number of pharmaceutical companies all support a number of prizes. This can include prizes for speciality essays for example from Arthritis Research UK.

Grants

Once you've been awarded a grant you should shout about it! Grants are competitively awarded and therefore demonstrate your potential for a career in academic medicine. Give the code for the grant, dates, and the awarding body and make it prominent.

You may have performed research as part of somebody else's grant. This would be something to put here, with an explanation of your role. A detailed account should be given within the 'research' part of the CV.

Research history

There are many opportunities to become involved in research during your undergraduate years and during your clinical training. Get involved early, even if you are unsure of your final career path. Explain what you did (briefly) in your CV.

Intercalated degrees

Doing an intercalated degree will provide ample opportunities to conduct research. We would encourage you to perform a laboratory- or research-based dissertation project rather than a library project. This will be an excellent exposure to the methodology of research and what it involves. The content of your individual project is less important, rather it is what you learned and the transferable skills that you can apply.

Clinical research

Other research opportunities can exist during early clinical training in helping with ongoing departmental studies or those of your consultants or higher trainees. For example, as a FY doctor you could volunteer to perform data trawls or input raw clinical data into databases. You may be involved in recruiting patients into studies and gaining their consent: an essential skill to emphasise.

Higher degrees

You may have produced some research as part of an MSc and this should be emphasised here. Clearly if you have done an MD or PhD you will have lots of information to fill this space!

Current projects

If you have a project currently on the go, you should describe it in detail, particularly any funding attached to the project and the publications and presentations it has generated. You should cover the purpose of the work and your attraction to it. Include what you have done specifically and its value to the field and how it relates to current knowledge. Acknowledge limitations and what needs to be done next. While some suggest you present your entire abstract, this is not practical and any publications are likely to be downloaded anyway (see Example 5.4).

Example 5.4

Clinical research
COIN Trial
November 2006 to February 2007
During my Oncology SHO post at St Elsewhere's, I actively recruited ward patients to the COIN Trial, which assessed the role of cetuximab in the

treatment of metastatic bowel malignancy. Patients were identified during consultant ward rounds, and I explained the trial process, the role of randomisation and value of participating in studies. I received training in obtaining consent. I liaised with the trial co-ordinator to organise trial assessments and investigations.

Laboratory research
Oligodendrocytes in rat models of ischaemic cerebral injury
October 2000–June 2001

Laboratory-based research project performed during intercalated BSc in Neuroscience. I conducted a detailed literature review on rat models of cerebral ischaemia, specifically the role of oligodendrocytes. Using this information, I collaborated with a PhD student to design and develop a protocol to study *in vitro* oligodendrocytes using chemically induced ischaemia. I then led this research project. I learnt *in vitro* experimental techniques, including performing biochemical assays, cell culture and electron microscopy. I gained skills in time management, animal handling and dissection as well as handling a large amount of computerised data.

The work was funded by the Cabol award from the Neuroscientist's Society, which was won in open competition. I was awarded a prize by the University of Cardiff for my dissertation. The findings were published in a peer-reviewed journal.

Key points
- You should emphasise:
    - Aims of the research and whether achieved
    - Your research techniques
    - What practical skills you gained
    - How your research added to your overall knowledge and skill mix
    - Your responsibilities in the project
    - The publications arising from it
    - Any posters, abstracts or presentations

Publications

All publications are important. Those in peer-reviewed journals should be listed before those in non-peer-reviewed journals and invited submissions (see Example 5.5). If you have contributed to a book then also place this here. Letters to journals are also helpful in demonstrating your interest in the field and that you are prepared to get involved. In general use reverse chronological order. Use the Vancouver citation style and give Pubmed numbers if available. Remember the reader of your CV is likely to look these papers up, so ensure everything you put is accurate. Put your name in bold to emphasise your role. Do not change the author order.

Example 5.5

Original research papers

Cole KC, **David LA**, Patel G. Multiple ligand binding sites are blocked by KA11223 in a dose dependent manner. *Br J Pharmacol* 2008;331:255–8

Abstracts

Cole KC, **David LA**, Patel G. KA11223 is a novel antagonist of cerebral glutamate receptors in rats. *J Neuroscience* 2007;877:192P

Case reports

David LA, Satayam M, Villa D. Total skin eruption following clopidogrel administration. *Journal of Case Reports* 2010; published online: JCR2010.1.10.131. PMID:18656098

Presentations

Whilst you may have given many presentations at your local hospital, supervisors are looking for presentations of original work at national and international conferences. This can include audits presented. You may have presented your work as a poster at such a meeting and this should be included (Example 5.6). If you contributed to someone else's poster, your name should be listed as an author and can be listed here.

Example 5.6

Poster presentations

Cole KC, **David LA**, Patel G. KA11223 is a novel antagonist of cerebral glutamate receptors in rats. *Brain* 2009, Shanghai (*international conference*)

Local presentation

David LA, Joshi K. Introduction of clerking proforma: results of a 6 month audit. St Elsewhere's Hospital, Clinical Governance Day, July 2009

Courses attended

There are a large number of courses available for everything you can think of. In themselves they do not count for a great deal. After all, the majority are a passive experience for you. However, you will be expected to attend specific courses on how to teach others, management skills and some courses key for your subspeciality (Example 5.7). For example, cardiologists can attend courses on echocardiography and for respiratory physicians, bronchoscopy courses. List these in reverse-chronological order. Some universities deliver short courses on research methodology and are worth pursuing.

Example 5.7

| 2007 | Teaching the Teachers | Royal College of Physicians |

4-week modular course providing training on teaching skills. I have deployed my knowledge in all subsequent undergraduate teaching

| 2006 | Surgical Skills for Juniors | University of Keele |

1-day practical skills course that was essential for my SHO posts at St Elsewhere's

In clinical CVs, you may put your advanced life support (ALS) and basic life support (BLS) training courses here, and although less important in an academic CV still should be included if space permits. Up-to-date ALS certification (or paediatric or neonatal) may be an essential criterion for ACF posts at higher level (e.g. ST3 in medical specialities).

Audit

Audit, quality improvement and service development are an essential component of clinical work and are common interview questions. You may even gain publications from your audits. However, be clear in your definitions of audit and research. Audit of course assesses current clinical practice against some standard (Example 5.8), whereas research asks novel questions about what might be the best approach or treatment, causes or effects.

List audits in reverse chronological order with their dates, title and a brief description. Again, the focus should be on what you learnt and the transferable skills you gained. The more audits you have, the less you should write about them. It is absolutely essential that you have, and state that you have, closed the audit cycle. Audits that are not closed are less useful and less well rated than those which have been. If it is too soon to close the audit cycle, then say so! Give your estimated time to closure and how it will be done. You should aim to perform one sizeable audit each year. Audits provide ample opportunities to demonstrate key skills essential to conducting research. You must be organised, be able to perform literature searches, collect and report data in a systematic way and interpret your findings. You need to be autonomous, focused and adaptable to answer the key question. Equally, you need time management and teamworking skills. All of these skills are transferable, especially to research, and should be emphasised.

Example 5.8

Audit into thromboprophylaxis use on the acute oncology wards at St Elsewhere:

- I identified that NHS targets on the use of low-molecular-weight heparin and stockings were not being reached in high-risk patients at St Elsewhere's Hospital. I retrieved trust and NICE guidelines that established the 'standard'. I designed an audit proforma. I coordinated with the audit office

- I conducted a prospective audit on the acute oncology wards for 3 months. 150 distinct patient episodes were recorded. Only 52% of patients had thromboembolic risk scores completed and only 30% were receiving thromboprophylaxis of any kind. Only 4% had contraindications to thromboprophylaxis
- Audit findings were presented to the department and the local Clinical Governance meeting. I implemented change to trust policy by writing new guidelines and by introducing a warning sticker attached to all drug charts. Training was delivered to junior doctors by a consultant colleague
- Repeat audit performed after 6 months showed an increase to 60% use of thromboprophylaxis. A further round of education is being delivered currently
- I specifically learnt the importance of presenting the data in a sensitive way to engender cooperation in a blame-free environment. I learnt to manage support staff to aid data collection and to use spreadsheets to collect and analyse the data

Teaching

Teaching others is an essential part of a doctor's role, especially an academic, and you will be expected to have delivered teaching to undergraduate medical students, more junior colleagues and members of the multidisciplinary team at almost any level of academic application. You should also have had specific training on how to teach certainly above core training levels, and ideally some training even earlier, and you should actively seek written feedback to know how to improve your teaching. The extent to which you will have done all this will depend on your seniority and level of training.

Key points

Within the teaching section comment on:

- Formal lectures
- Formal clinical teaching
- Informal teaching
- Teaching outside of medicine
- Your training for teaching

Your teaching may predominantly be informal bedside teaching. If that is the case, take the opportunity to arrange a series of tutorials for your local undergraduates. Make some feedback forms and distribute them during the session. You can rapidly develop a good reputation if you do this well and this looks golden on your CV and portfolio. You may have been fortunate enough to give formal teaching at your local university or other institute. If so, it is worth stating how this opportunity came about. For example, state if you were specifically invited to give the talks or if it formed part of your post. More senior individuals will have delivered teaching at a postgraduate level. You may also have delivered teaching in other ways, such as making a website or writing a book.

Career summary

All CVs will have a career summary. For an academic CV you do not need to give a detailed description of each post and what your tasks were. List your posts in reverse chronological order. Any gaps in your career should be accounted for. Your speciality of choice can be highlighted using bold to show the amount of experience you have in it. Example 5.9 presents one such summary.

Example 5.9

Oct 09	ST4: **Respiratory Medicine**	Elsewhere Hospital, London	Dr Grant
Oct 08	ST3: **Respiratory Medicine**	Nowhere NHS Trust, London	Dr Lesley
Aug 08	LAT: **Respiratory Medicine**	Overthere NHS Trust, Bristol	Dr Smith

Aug 06–08
        Core Medical Training   University Hospital, Leeds   Dr Evans
        ST2: Cardiology, Oncology, Neurology
        ST1: **Respiratory**, A&E, Renal Medicine

Aug 05–06
        FY2   Glenside Hospital, Cumbria Dr Probert
        FY2: General Practice, A&E, **Respiratory**

Aug 04–05
        FY1   Otherside Hospital, Cumbria Mr El-Dar
        FY1: Vascular surgery, cardiology, urology

Personal statement

You may wish to place this at the beginning of your CV. Essentially it is a brief statement of your aspirations and what you intend to do to achieve them (Example 5.10). This will help confirm you as an individual with your own thoughts and ideas. Your supervisor may have other ideas however, but at least you can show you have your own drivers and ambition. Do not copy one off the Internet!

Example 5.10

I am a vascular surgery ST5 with a special interest in inflammatory cell distribution in unstable atheroma present in large arteries. In particular I am interested in the basic biology of the inflammatory process and the role of cytokine switching. My intention is to pursue an academic career in vascular biology with a focus on cytokines. In the short term I will undertake a PhD in this field. My long-term goal is to lead a research group as a reader and then as a professor of vascular biology, while working as a vascular surgeon.

You should spend time perfecting your CV and addressing any gaps to create a well-rounded CV. Do not leave it until the last minute. You should add to your CV as you gain new achievements. Remember that your CV is a story of your career and a 'sales pitch' that distinguishes you from the crowd. It is a platform from which you can launch new projects, generate discussions at interview and bring in job opportunities. Look again at your CV and modify it so you achieve *that* post, project or funding.

Key points – CV summary

- Target your CV to the individual post or academic position you are applying for; analyse the job description and make sure your CV clearly meets the 'essential' and 'desired' criteria
- Use clear presentation and consistent fonts and font sizes
- Use bullet points and short sentences
- Emphasise your contribution, what you learnt and how you do and will apply it
- Use Vancouver style for your publications
- Avoid acronyms and minimise jargon

Academic application and interview

Philip J Smith
Sukhjinder S Nijjer
Jeremy B Levy
Jasdeep K Gill

Applying for academic training posts – academic clinical fellowship (ACF) or clinical lectureship (CL) or others – can seem to be a 'leap of faith' at times, with applications and interviews for such posts being distinct from the mainstream speciality job selection process. However, common themes are repeated during the academic application/interview process across the specialities, with the speciality-specific questions being entwined with questions relating to the applicant's prior academic career and achievements, their current career plans and aims, and academic plans for the future. The aim is to identify those who will be most capable of balancing the stresses and strains of an academic career with the clinical demands of these posts, and those most likely to become high-quality research active academic clinicians and ultimately senior lecturers or professors!

How and when to apply for academic training

The applications for ACF and CL placements are organised through local deaneries under the aegis of the National Institute for Health Research Trainees Co-ordinating Centre (NIHRTCC, www.nihrtcc.nhs.uk). The NIHRTCC determines the number of posts available at any time depending on the funding available and a competitive process between universities and specialities to win such posts. Advertisements are found on the deanery websites usually at least a few weeks in advance of the opening date for applications.

Application to posts occurs in two phases. Round 1 opens usually in October or November of each year and is typically when the majority of available academic posts are advertised and consequently filled if suitable candidates are found.

For trainees applying for an ACF the timing of these advertisements is deliberate to allow the shortlisting and interview processes for such a post not to impact on potential applications for conventional (non-academic) speciality training posts (which usually start after December). Even if you are not successful in obtaining an academic training post you can still apply for a conventional post, although you obviously can't accept both! Round 2 of applications opens once the previous round has closed, and includes posts not filled during the previous round; this may also include a few additional posts in some specialties. Round 2 opening and closing can be unpredictable so it is important to pay attention to the deanery websites so not to miss opportunities. If posts remain unfilled they can be advertised later in the year. Keep watching out or ask directly the academic lead for the programme you are interested in applying for; their names and contact details are on the NIHR and deanery websites.

Key points

- If you are considering submitting an application for an academic post, think ahead, visit your deanery website or contact the NIHRTCC.
- Ask around – speak to other academic trainees on the pros and cons of applying for particular academic posts.

Before starting – making the most of what you have

The application form is the first hurdle you must leap to get the all-important interview, so it must be right. No doubt if you are reading this book and seriously contemplating an academic career, you will recognise by now that preparation and organisation way in advance of the submission is essential.

To prepare thoroughly for the application (and also the interview) there are a number of steps that can help organise your thoughts and plans so nothing is omitted:

- ★ Sit down and update your curriculum vitae (CV) – note down your career achievements, think about the research you have done and write a short summary of your experiences.
- ★ Be realistic – these posts may be very competitive, and to avoid any disappointment ensure you meet all the requirements before applying.
- ★ Read the personal specification and the scoring sheet before starting – you can pick out areas where you are weaker and there may be time to rectify this.
- ★ Have it clear in your mind why you are applying for the post, what the post involves and what your end goals are.
- ★ Research the areas that you have an interest in – visit potential supervisors, make contacts, make it known that you are considering an academic career – people are usually helpful.
- ★ Arrange a meeting with your supervisor to review your application and let others read it too – they may spot gaps you have overlooked.

★ Sell yourself! This is no time to keep to yourself the two *Nature* publications you have or be shy about your first-name paper in the *Lancet!!*

Application scoring criteria

Examples of the ACF and CL applications can be found on the deanery websites, with standardised graded scoring guidelines in use by deaneries to help distinguish between candidates. An applicant must meet the specified essential entry criteria for the post as stated on the application form and person specification. This varies depending on the level of entry into academic training. For example, to be able to apply for ST3 ACF posts evidence of Foundation competencies, achievement of core speciality training competencies, relevant Royal College membership exam success (e.g. MRCP), and at least 24 months' experience in core speciality training is necessary.

Beware!

You must ensure you are eligible for the post before you apply or else your application will be immediately rejected.

Academic clinical fellowship: Application scoring

Applications are increasingly web based rather than using downloaded forms for completing and returning by email or hard copies. They will remain based on the same principles and details as described below even if the format changes. The precise scores can also vary between application forms in different specialties or regions or level of application, and the examples given here will allow you to judge relative importance.

Once it is clear that a candidate meets the entry criteria they are further assessed on specified selection criteria and given a maximum score out of 36 (this score can vary by post, level, speciality and deanery), and then all applicants ranked against each other to decide who gets shortlisted for interview.

A typical application form would be scored in the following way:

1 Essential selection criteria (maximum score of 14 points).
   Clinical experience (assessed from specific sections of the form) is
      scored from 0 points = no evidence of relevant clinical experience to
      3 points = evidence of above average clinical experience.
   Academic experience (assessed from specific sections of the form) is
      scored from 0 points = no evidence of relevant academic experience to
      3 points = evidence of above average academic experience.
   Commitment to a clinical academic career (assessed from specific sections
      of the form) is scored from 0 points = no evidence of commitment to this

career path to 4 points = ample, clear and comprehensive evidence of commitment.

Language skills (assessed from all aspects of the form) is scored from 0 points = no evidence of competence in written English to 2 points = clear and concise use of appropriate written English.

Reasoned/analytical approach (assessed from all aspects of the form) is scored from 0 points = no evidence of reasoned/analytical approach to applying for the post in completing the form to 2 points = provides evidence throughout of reasons for applying, and clearly links experience to the post being applied for.

Note: Scoring zero in any essential criteria will usually lead to an automatic rejection of an application.

2 Desirable selection criteria (maximum score of 22).

Degrees (in some applications only one is marked).

BA or BSc	0 points = None	3 points = 1st class
MSc or MRes	0 points = None	3 points = Distinction
PhD or MD	0 points = None	3 points = Awarded

Undergraduate or postgraduate prizes – This ranges from 0 points for no prizes to 2 points for three or more prizes or one very prestigious prize such as a University Gold Medal.

Honours/distinctions – This ranges from 0 points for no honours/distinctions to 2 points for three or more honours/distinctions.

Teaching experience – Those with no teaching role/experience are scored 0 points, while those with a formal role receiving 2 points.

Extra-curricular activities – Zero points for no evidence of any additional activities and 2 points for activities relevant to a clinical academic career in that speciality.

Scientific publications – For those candidates with four or more publications as a major author including at least one in a leading journal for the speciality or other major journal, the maximum score is 4 points. Again, there is a reduction in points awarded in a graded fashion, with no points for no publications!

Scientific presentations – Presentation at an international meeting achieves a maximum total of 3 points, with 0 points if no evidence of presentations is provided.

Key academic achievements – Those deemed by shortlisters to have outstanding evidence of academic achievement are scored 4 points, whereas no evidence of academic potential is given 0 points.

Useful information

Shortlisters are advised that the scores from the desired criteria must be viewed in the context of the applicant's level and the point at which they are attempting to apply for an academic number

▦ Academic clinical fellowship: Application form

The application form itself is divided up into sections, with the first few sections allowing the applicant to simply list their career path and highlights to date in the following areas:

- Present and previous employment.
- Additional experience, training, courses and extracurricular achievements relevant to this speciality.
- Professional qualifications.
- Academic achievements.
  - Prizes, or other academic distinctions
  - Publications
  - Presentations/posters.

The remaining sections of the application form are subdivided into 'white space answers', inviting the applicant to write about their research and academic experience within a strict word limit – usually between 150–250 words. Below are some worked examples of typical application questions (these are examples of course and should not be copied verbatim nor used as templates but give a flavour of the information being sought by shortlisters and interviewers).

Research experience and academic career plans

"Please give brief details of all research projects and/or relevant research experience that you have undertaken or are undertaking, including methods used. Indicate your level of involvement and your exact role in the research team (up to 150 words)"

> *"I have conducted two major research projects in which I have acted as lead investigator:*
> - *I designed and developed the 'Cystic Fibrosis Health Locus of Control' scale for children, testing the validity and test/re-test reliability of the scale against an already valid generic locus of control scale. Children with cystic fibrosis were asked to complete both scales, with the scores of each scale being analysed to test the validity of the new scale*
> - *As part of the St Elsewhere's Infection Control group I instigated an investigation into whether there was any association between the length of time a peripherally inserted central catheter (PICC) line was left in situ and bacteraemia rates in oncology patients*
> *In both projects, I collected the data, co-ordinated its analysis and also worked as part of a multidisciplinary research team. The successful completion of these projects has led to two publications in peer-reviewed journals". (146 words)*

"Please describe in more detail one of the research projects above" (up to 150 words)

"Whilst working at St Elsewhere's Hospital, I expressed my interest in infectious diseases and was invited to be the lead researcher testing the hypothesis that the length of time that a PICC line was in situ was associated with bacteraemia rates in oncology patients.

Using the data of over 300 patients collected by the St Elsewhere's study group, I developed a proforma to collect the data, collated it and then analysed this using non-parametrics. A team of senior researchers and clinicians supported me. The results suggested a statistically significant relationship between length of time of PICC line insertion and rates of bacteraemia in this cohort of immunocompromised patients. These results supported previous clinical research findings that poor PICC line care predisposed patients to increased risk of bacteraemia over use of conventional venous access.

This study was presented at 21st European Society of Oncology Conference in Paris 2008". (148 words)

"Please state why you want this particular academic clinical fellowship, indicating your medium- and long-term career goals in relation to an academic career in this speciality area" (up to 150 words)

"I have always been interested in following an academic career path, having thoroughly enjoyed undertaking my two previous research projects. During my ACF post I would like to pursue this interest further by combining my clinical specialist registrar training with some further research projects. I would utilise my time to gain some generic research science skills and to identify an area of interest that I may then develop to obtain a higher degree such as a PhD, after applying for funding from the Wellcome Trust or the MRC.

I am committed to a continuing career in academic surgery and hope that this ACF post will be the first step on the path to becoming a clinical lecturer and eventually an independent investigator in this field". (125 words)

"How will this training programme and your previous training and experience help you meet your career objectives? What are your reasons for applying to this training programme"? (up to 250 words)

"I have successfully completed my core medical training rotation and am a clinically competent speciality trainee with a range of clinical and communication skills. I have completed several cardiology posts and my exposure to different presentations of cardiology problems in different patient groups has developed my interest in this speciality.

I am fully committed to cardiology and post MRCP have sought out opportunities to learn how to perform basic echocardiograms. I have developed my organisational and IT skills through research and audits, and presented twice internationally on subjects related to cardiology:

- *'The role of calcium channel mutations in long QT syndrome' (Madrid 2009).*
- *My audit on the 'Management of acute coronary syndrome in a central London tertiary centre' (Rome 2008).*

Since writing a review on the 'Methods of undergraduate teaching in medical school' I have continued to develop an interest in medical education. As an associate Royal College of Physicians tutor, I formally teach medical students on a regular basis, at the bedside and on ward rounds. The TIPS course for clinical teachers has reinforced these skills.

I hope this academic training programme will enable me to pursue my passion for cardiology, engaging in research and audit in this area and enabling me to dedicate more time to teaching. I hope that I will then be well placed to obtain research funding to pursue a higher research degree with the ultimate aim to eventually become an independent investigator in my own right in the future". (248 words)

The 'white space answers' can be frustrating to write and word appropriately. However it is crucial that time is taken on these sections to ensure that you are able to articulate your past academic and non-academic achievements, clinical training, as well as your future career intentions so you score highly enough to be shortlisted.

Clinical lectureship: Application scoring

For a clinical lectureship (CL) post a typical application form has a slightly different scoring system with scores given out of 50, and the range for each assessed area being from 0 to a maximum of 2. Again this can vary by deanery and speciality. The minimum score to be considered for shortlisting in this circumstance is 20, with the scores of all candidates being ranked to determine who is ultimately shortlisted. A score of 0 within the essential criteria means the candidate cannot be shortlisted.

The areas that are normally assessed on the application form (and at interview) are summarised in Table 6.1. Some of these are in fact only scored at the interview itself.

Clinical lectureship: Application form

Some applicants for a CL will have never applied for a training fellowship before or have an academic training number (from an ACF post for example). However all will have significant clinical and research training experience if applying for such posts. There is no need to have been in ACF post to apply for a CL post. Predictably the CL application form is even more detailed, and contains more 'white space' answers covering some additional sections not covered in the ACF application form. As reflected in the typical CL scoring, each of these sections is very important as valuable points are associated with them. In a similar vein to the ACF application, the candidate is asked to list their employment history, publications, posters, conferences attended, as well as awards, achievements and prizes.

Table 6.1: Essential and desirable criteria when applying for a CL

Essential	Desirable
PhD, MD (original research)	Intercalated BSc, BA, MSc
Evidence of experience of and active participation in audit	Other degrees, qualifications
Experience of working in multiprofessional teams	Academic prizes and honours
Knowledge of how to obtain informed consent	Experience in a broad range of acute and chronic speciality settings
Communication and interpersonal skills	Additional training and experience in wider speciality
Demonstrates drive and initiative	Appropriate progression of career
Clarity of career aspirations	Management/financial awareness, experience of committee work, understanding of the NHS, clinical governance and resource constraints with specific reference to the delivery of speciality services
Understanding of how academic training will provide opportunities for career development	Ability to produce legible notes
Potential for development as a clinical academic in research	Demonstrates the ability to write scientific papers in a clear and organised fashion
Research experience	Enthusiasm for teaching, exposure to different groups/teaching methods
Research plans	Teaching the Teachers course
Publications in peer-reviewed journals	
Publications in other journals	
Presentations	
Experience of teaching	

Useful information

You do not have to answer each of these questions in continuous prose – bullet points are acceptable and will help to articulate what you want to say concisely.

Below are a number of worked examples of how to answer the 'white space' questions. Again these are just examples to show what you might include and not meant to be used as templates! Your answer should be individual to you and reflect the work you have done.

Clinical experience

"Please give details of your clinical experience that would be of particular use in this post"

- *"I have received excellent medical training to date, including on the St Elsewhere's Medical SHO rotation.*
- *4 years' clinical experience of oncology patient management – both in the inpatient and outpatient settings.*

- *Excellent experience in managing a wide range of tumour types – managing rare tumours and paediatric malignancies as part of a multidisciplinary team.*
- *Wide experience of the management of acute medical and oncological emergencies while on call.*
- *Involvement in ongoing clinical trials – actively enrolling, consenting and managing patients who are appropriate for such trials. In addition, I have experience of reporting serious adverse events related to chemotherapy as well as communicating with the sponsor and principal investigator.*
- *Excellent communication skills and organisational ability, and ability to lead a multidisciplinary team and junior medical staff.*
- *Wide range of clinical skills including central line insertion, chest drain insertion, abdominal paracentesis, managing non-invasive ventilation and performing lumbar punctures.*
- *Good Clinical Practice certified.*
- *Advanced Life Support certified.*
- *Excellent organisational and communication skills".*

"Summarise your clinical experience and skills in respiratory medicine" (maximum 100 words)

(An alternative question may be): "Please describe the experience you have gained in the management of unselected medical emergencies, indicating the most senior level of responsibility you have held during the medical take"

"I have been a respiratory trainee for 3 years and am a competent, confident clinician with a wealth of experience of caring for patients, including managing those requiring invasive or non-invasive ventilation, as well as dealing with patients with end-stage lung disease. I am able to lead medical on-calls confidently, prioritising plans on the basis of clinical need. I have performed over 400 diagnostic bronchoscopies and over 100 therapeutic endoscopy procedures. I am competent in performing lung biopsies and chest drain insertion. I communicate effectively with patients and colleagues alike, as well as having excellent organisational skills".

"Please indicate any additional skills that you would bring to this appointment"

- *"Intensive care experience as part of my clinical training.*
- *Experience of consenting, recruiting and performing clinical trials.*
- *Experience of different research methodologies – conducting a successful research project during my MRC-funded PhD.*
- *A good working relationship with colleagues and other members of the multidisciplinary team – being able to lead meetings when appropriate.*
- *Extensive experience of formal teaching as an associate Royal College of Physicians tutor and running successful MRCP PACES courses.*

- *Experience of ethics applications, the ability to successfully gain research funding, as well as academic ability in writing high-impact research papers and critical appraisal of other research papers.*
- *Competent information technology (IT) and presentational skills".*

Audit

"Please describe your experience of clinical audit. Indicate clearly your own level of involvement"

- *"I have been actively involved in audit projects as part of ongoing clinical governance since qualifying in 2000. I have acted as clinical lead for a number of audit projects on subjects including: 'The management of acute coronary syndromes' in A&E; 'The prescription of cholesterol-lowering medications post myocardial infarction' management, as well as 'Audit of infective complications post pacemaker insertion' during my cardiology specialist training.*
- *I have also recently acted as a clinical lead for a multi-site audit of 'The management of cardiac patients post emergency percutaneous coronary intervention'. The results of this audit are currently being collated and analysed.*
- *I have completed the 'audit cycle' related to an audit on – 'The prescription of beta blockers for patients with left ventricular failure' – in my previous post, leading to a change in clinical practice. I was responsible for the data collection, analysis and report writing".*

Management skills

A number of questions have been used to approach this important area, often related to managing teams both inside and outside of work. These include:

"Please describe any experience of managing people. You may give examples from both inside and outside medicine"

"Please describe your experience of working in an effective team and how you saw your role. You may give examples from inside or outside medicine"

"Please describe your experience of managing resources. You may give examples from both inside and outside medicine"

"Please describe the strengths and weaknesses of working in a multidisciplinary team"

Strengths
- *Facilitates decision making and standardisation of care for all patients.*
- *Helps to reduce referral time.*

- *Obtain perspectives from many different health professionals.*
- *Supportive forum for difficult case discussion.*
- *Allows review of pathology and radiology.*

Weaknesses
- *Time consuming.*
- *Difficult for all members to be present at all meetings.*
- *Requires investment of resources to support the multidisciplinary team (MDT).*
- *Can lead to unnecessary referrals if essential clinical information is not known for each patient".*

Miscellaneous questions

The following are typical questions on the application form:

"Please indicate your level of familiarity with IT"

This question is self-explanatory and familiarity with IT will vary between applicants – although a good working knowledge is clearly important.

"Please describe the last exchange you had with a patient when you needed informed consent"

"I am currently caring for a man with TB meningitis who is highly suspected to have HIV. This man recently presented to hospital with his wife confused and agitated at home, after returning from a trip to Kenya. On the ward his conscious level deteriorated, despite starting on appropriate anti-TB medications. Clinically this man had multiple hallmarks of profound immunosuppression. He therefore required aggressive treatment. However, the patient was deemed incompetent to provide informed consent. He was unable to process and retain the information given and so he was not able to consent for an HIV test initially. Furthermore, he was not able to understand the implications and consequences of the treatment. This was complicated further by the future requirement for his wife to be tested for HIV. Once the man had responded to the treatment given, and it was clear he had capacity to give informed consent, I discussed with him confidentially our clinical suspicions and he agreed to a HIV test. This was proven positive. With the support of the HIV multidisciplinary team he was counselled further and started on appropriate anti-retroviral treatment. Together with the multidisciplinary team, the patient and his wife were supported through this difficult time. Through my actions, the patient gave full informed consent to this test without breaking his confidentiality at any time".

"In approximately 150 words discuss what you think is currently the most important issue in medical oncology"

"The challenge of improving survival rates is one of the most important issues for oncologists at present. Recently, the United States 'Annual Report to the

Nation' showed that large improvements in survival rates have been seen in cancers of the colon, prostate and breast. There are many conditions however where prognosis remains poor and progress has been slow in development of new treatments such as in cancers of the lung and pancreas. One of the ongoing challenges for medical oncologists is to work with colleagues in the oncology multidisciplinary team to tackle this issue. Huge benefits have been seen recently with targeted therapies against tumours such as renal cell carcinomas that have contributed significantly to improved survival rates. The role of such therapies in the context of solid tumours and in the adjuvant setting may be the direction into which medical oncologists can make the most difference". (147 words)

Other achievements

A range of personal skills is assessed on the CL application forms, which have been identified as being particularly important in successful practitioners. Each skill requires a succinct answer where applicants can draw on experiences both inside and outside of work, to answer these questions.

Communication and interpersonal skills

"In approximately 150 words describe the most challenging situation you have ever been in and how you dealt with this"

"In Accident and Emergency as the paediatric registrar on call, I have been constantly challenged by the cases presenting to hospital. Recently, a 4-year-old child was admitted unconscious with a blood glucose reading of less than 1. The child's mother gave an inconsistent history, informing the admitting team that she had found her child on the floor. His grandmother was diabetic, and there was a needle mark on the child's body. I was concerned that this was non-accidental injury. After successfully resuscitating the child as my first priority, I explained to the mother that her child needed to be admitted to hospital for further observation and investigation. I informed the consultant, social worker, and nursing staff about my concerns. After organic causes were excluded, as a team we investigated the possibility of fabricated illness to ensure the child's safety and well being, while maintaining a rapport with the mother". (147 words)

Initiative

"In approximately 150 words please give an example that best illustrates your drive and initiative"

"I singlehandedly developed, and continue to manage an MRCP PACES course at St Elsewhere's hospital, which runs three times a year, every night for a month. This provides clinical teaching to speciality trainees attempting to sit their PACES examinations. Each examination station is covered during the course, with representatives from each speciality on the faculty. As well as

teaching on the course, I also recruit all the clinical tutors for the course, from professors through to specialist registrars. The course has been highly successful, gaining excellent feedback from candidates and tutors alike, demonstrating my strong organisational skills. With the course entering its third year, it boasts a pass rate from attendees of greater than 80%. As the course director, I have been awarded the 'Chairman's Medal' for innovation and initiative, as well as being made an associate Royal College of Physicians tutor". (144 words)

Demonstrating potential

"Explain how you have developed your interest in becoming an academic medical specialist and how this illustrates your potential for the development of a career in research"

"Since medical school, I have tried to develop my academic career, gaining a first-class intercalated BSc in Immunology, and producing a number of peer-reviewed publications during this time. I have applied this knowledge to my clinical duties and pursued my interest in defective immunity by pursuing a career in HIV medicine. While in the junior years of my medical training I continued to expand my knowledge in this area by working within Professor X's laboratory in my spare time, to build upon my previous experimental work. After obtaining my Royal College membership exams and national training number in this speciality area, I gained a Wellcome Trust Clinical Research Training Fellowship to work in Tanzania to complete a 3-year PhD, investigating the 'Mechanisms of HIV-associated immune reconstitution syndrome'. I successfully completed this, publishing more than eight peer-reviewed papers.

Despite this, I feel there are many unanswered hypotheses and questions in this area of research, which is so clinically relevant in the advent of increasing anti-retroviral use across the globe. I want to pursue my academic career and hope to obtain a clinical lectureship so I can combine my experimental work with exposure to immunodeficient patients in clinics and hospital to bring context to my work.

Throughout my career, I have also been actively involved in audit projects and have continued to gain experience of teaching at all levels.

Based on my track record in academic medicine and my future research plans, I feel I am well positioned to combine my specialist training with further research into this exciting area, and hope this will propel me ultimately into becoming an independent investigator".

Academic achievements

All candidates will be asked about the details of their research experience (whether past or in progress) as well as indicating their involvement. This is difficult to demonstrate in a worked example, but it is critical that you demonstrate clearly and succinctly the periods of time you have been involved in scientific research. A suggested format for this could be:

* State the dates in which the research has occurred.
* The research qualification obtained (e.g. PhD).
* The funding body or fellowship obtained for the research (e.g. Medical Research Council, Wellcome Trust).
* The laboratory/department/hospital/university in which you were based.
* Your supervisor's name and speciality area.
* Name of research project.
* A brief description of actual research and its conclusions/outcomes.

Again candidates will be asked to outline plans for research in the CL. This needs to contain the following factors:

* Be clear and concise.
* Demonstrate a commitment to an academic career in that speciality.
* Have clear questions and outcomes.
* Have an idea of where you want to base yourself, collaborate with and who your mentor will be – and what are the benefits of you working there.
* Relevance to the speciality in which the post is.
* Have clear timeframes and be realistic in view of time spent in clinical work and in academic time.

Teaching

In contrast to the ACF application form, evidence of involvement in teaching is crucial and it's an area in which you can pick up 'easier' marks. For example, you will be asked to list your experience of teaching and also state if you have been on any Teaching the Teachers courses. If you haven't then it may be worth correcting this so you don't miss out on crucial points in the application process!

Formal research training

This is the part of the application form where you can demonstrate the research skills you have developed. This will be different depending on whether you have worked in a laboratory before, done purely clinical research, or worked with animals/humans.

An example is as follows:

> *"During my intercalated BSc and then MRC CTF-funded PhD, I received training in the following:*
> * *PCR, Western blotting, tissue culture, ELISA, RNA purification and the use of micro arrays*
> * *Use of radioactivity within the laboratory*
> * *Critical appraisal of research papers*
> * *How to write a research paper*
> * *Statistical analysis*

- *Good Clinical Practice*
- *Presentation skills"*

Aims and career objectives

This section should be a clear statement of intent as to why you are applying for this post and what you hope to achieve, for example:

> "I am currently on the St Elsewhere's surgical training rotation with a surgical national training number and am fully committed to a career in academic surgery. I thoroughly enjoyed my previous research experiences and would like to extend upon the work I performed in my PhD while at the same time continue with my clinical training.
>
> In this post, I hope to continue my research into the molecular and environmental mechanisms involved in the development of colorectal carcinoma, using my clinical and academic acumen to direct the focus of my research. I hope to be able to contribute towards the understanding of the pathogenesis of this complex malignancy. I believe that developing this understanding and using my generic research skills will be vital for my development as a clinical academic surgeon. Based on my previous academic track record and continued commitment to academia, I hope I will be a strong candidate for this clinical lectureship position".

Interests, other skills and achievements outside medicine

A tricky section! You feel you have to put something to demonstrate that you are a well-rounded individual, but at the same time you don't want to undo the image you have portrayed of yourself in the rest of the application! Choose what you decide to put down carefully. In the end it does not usually count for anything but may provide a focus for a brief discussion at the interview or make you stand out.

Any additional information relevant to this application

If you have already applied for grants or funding, or have a research proposal put them within this section – it further demonstrates initiative and that you are 'ready to go' once you are in post. But don't just repeat material elsewhere on the application form.

Key points

- Read the person specification attached to the application form
- If there is a score sheet attached to the form then read it. Score your application yourself, and more importantly get others to score it too!
- Ensure you can score highly in all sections of the form so you are shortlisted – especially the essential criteria!
- Plan way ahead when completing these forms and don't submit at the very last moment

- Use your CV as a guide so you don't miss anything vital off that could give you the extra vital points
- Make sure you don't miss out on the easy marks by poor spelling and punctuation!

Surviving the interview

If you get an interview you have done incredibly well. However, the same level of preparation and planning is required for this next hurdle. Remember that the interviewers will expect you to know about whatever you have put down on your application form, in detail. They will also question you about clinical scenarios within that speciality, so you need to be on your toes!

The interview itself normally consists of three sections lasting 30 minutes for an ACF interview, and slightly longer for CLs. The questions asked are linked to the person specification, with questions related to both the clinical and academic components of the post. Often one 'station' or section of the interview will be clinical especially for an ACF post to ensure you are suitable to train clinically in that speciality. If you were to fail this or demonstrate such poor performance then this would over-ride any academic excellence.

The three main academic areas assessed are:

* Knowledge and achievements.
* Scientific publications and presentations, and future academic plans.
* Communication skills.

Interviewers are typically taken from the institutions where the posts are available, with normally a 'lay observer', a deanery/speciality training programme director and an academic from another university being present. The scales shown as Table 6.2 are usually used by interviewers to score candidates.

Table 6.2: Scoring the candidate in interview

Score and justification	Criteria
0 No evidence	No evidence reported
1 Areas of concern	Limited number of specified positive behavioural indicators displayed
	Many negative indicators displayed, one or more decisively
2 Satisfactory	Satisfactory display of specified positive behavioural indicators
	Some negative indicators displayed, but not clearly
3 Good	Good display of specified positive behavioural indicators
	Few negative indicators displayed, but not clearly or decisively
4 Excellent	Excellent display of specified positive behavioural indicators (and possibly others)
	Little or no negative indicators displayed, and these considered minor in status

This scoring system can vary with scoring ranges between zero and two or five. The interview may take many forms with the order and phrasing of questions varying. However the overall structure will remain the same in any one interview session to ensure consistency between candidates, and with the same opening questions. In the CL interviews, questions may probe deeper into the research ideas, proposals and methodologies relating to the candidates proposals, whereas an ACF interview may aim to discover if the candidate has a real insight into what a clinical academic career involves – from ethical considerations to funding bodies. Both interviews could easily ask the candidate about probity-related issues and even clinical governance.

A typical interview may use a selection of these questions. Although these are certainly not all encompassing, these are some of the most commonly asked within clinical academic interviews.

Knowledge and achievements
Assessment made by interviewers

* The candidate demonstrates a general knowledge/broad interest in science and academic medicine and a knowledge of the clinical career pathway.
* The candidate demonstrates an acquisition of the level of knowledge and skills necessary for the completion of foundation/speciality/specialist training (to a specified level) with an emphasis on academic competencies.

Positive and negative indicators for general success at interview are given in Table 6.3.

Table 6.3: Indicators for success at interview

Positive indicators	Negative indicators
Provides clear and reasoned explanation for importance of academic medicine	Explanations/arguments are unclear or lack relevance
Shows accurate understanding of purpose and impact of academic medicine	Lacks understanding of purpose and impact of academic medicine
Shows awareness of basic principles of research methodology	Provides no evidence of personal experience of research or understanding of research methodology
Provides evidence of personal experience of research	Unable to link own experience to his/her arguments

Possible interview questions
* Why should doctors do research?
* Why choose this speciality?
* What interests you the most?
* What drives clinical academics?
* Why is academic medicine important?
* Why become an academic when the rewards are surely not as great as within the private sector?

* How has your clinical and research experience thus far helped you choose your career path?
* Tell me about your research, and specifically your role in it.
* What would you do differently with your research if you had to start again?
* What are the barriers to clinical research?
* Explain your understanding of clinical governance and your own involvement in this during your career to date.
* What is research governance and why is it important?
* Explain the importance of clinical audit.
* Tell me about an audit you have been involved in. What was your role and what was the outcome?
* What is the difference between clinical audit and research?
* Tell me about your understanding of risk management in institutions.
* What is the role of the National Institute of Clinical Excellence (NICE)/ National Patient Safety Agency (NPSA) in clinical research?
* Tell me about a NICE guideline you currently use in clinical practice.
* What paper has changed your clinical practice in the last few years?
* In your research proposal you have stated you are using this methodology; justify this.
* What ethical considerations relate to your research?
* How do you keep up to date with current research in your speciality?
* What are the major problems encountered in translational research?
* Tell me about an interesting paper you have recently read outside of your speciality.
* Explain how clinical trials are set up and the steps involved in this?
* Tell me how clinical researchers and scientists are funded.
* What is the greatest weakness you have in your academic career to date?
* What are the downsides to becoming a clinical academic in this speciality?
* Can you explain your research in one simple sentence?

Scientific publications and presentations

Assessment made by interviewers

* The candidate demonstrates clear career intentions as a clinical academic.
* The candidate demonstrates experience in research/publications/presentations.
* The candidate demonstrates potential for a career in educational/research through scientific publications and presentations (Table 6.4).

Possible interview questions

* What are your short-term career aims?
* What are you medium- to long-term career aims?
* Where do you see yourself in 5–10 years?
* If you were to get this post, how would it further your career progression?

* What are the barriers to becoming a career academic?
* Would obtaining an ACF/CL affect your career aims?
* Why apply to become an ACF/CL?
* What would you do with your ACF/CL?
* How do plan to spend you academic time?
* How would you balance your clinical and academic commitments?
* How would you judge whether your ACF/CL had been successful?
* What is your most important publication to date and why?
* Which of your publications has the highest impact and why?
* Tell me about your publications to date – what has been your role and what problems have you encountered?
* You were given this award/prize/honor – what was this for?
* What is your proudest academic achievement to date?
* When you presented this presentation, what were the main criticisms and questions?
* What inspired you to pursue an academic route?
* How do academics fit in within the structure of hospitals/institutions/universities?
* What experience of teaching do you have?
* What makes a good clinical academic tutor?
* Why should academics be interested in medical education?
* How would you incorporate teaching/medical education into your position?

Table 6.4: Indicators for success in reporting achievements and research at interview

Positive indicators	Negative indicators
Provides evidence of academic potential through presentations/publications/prizes and honours	Explanation of academic activities lacks clarity or relevance
Clear understanding of how research experience can contribute to development of a career as a clinical academic	Lacks understanding of how own experience can be built on in development of a career as a clinical academic
Shows how research interests are relevant to the ACF in this speciality	Fails to explain how own research interests can be aligned with the speciality

Communication skills

Assessment made by interviewers

* The candidate demonstrates clarity in written and spoken communication and capacity to adapt language as appropriate to the situation (Table 6.5).
* The candidate is able to build a rapport, listen, persuade and negotiate.
* The candidate demonstrates evidence of teamworking skills and leadership potential.

This may be assessed over the course of the whole interview rather than by using specific questions.

Table 6.5: Indicators relating to communication skills

Positive indicators	Negative indicators
Adjusts to style of questioning/responses as appropriate	Unable to adapt language/behaviour as needed
Able to express ideas to others clearly – written and spoken	Is patronising/domineering in communicating with others
Uses inventive language (e.g. humour/analogy) to explain	Use of language is too functional/narrow/technical
Uses active listening	Limited evidence of active listening
Makes effective use of non-verbal behaviour (voice, posture etc.)	Fails to engage others at non-verbal level

Miscellaneous questions

These questions are often used to judge attributes across several domains and to get candidates to think aloud:

* Tell me about an occasion when you needed to prioritise your time.
* Tell me about a clinical scenario where you had to prioritise patient care.
* How do you manage your time and deal with stress?
* Tell me about a situation where you had to deal with a challenging patient/difficult situation/difficult or struggling colleague.
* You are told on a ward round that a mistake has been made when dealing with a patient – how do you deal with this situation?
* Tell me about a time when you have made a mistake. How did you deal with this situation?
* Tell me about a time when you worked in a team – what was your role and responsibilities?
* What are the strengths and weaknesses of a MDT?
* Tell me about a time when you have had to act as a leader?
* What makes a good team?
* What makes a good leader?
* Describe a difficult case you have been involved in.
* Describe a time when your communication skills have made a difference to patient care.
* Tell me about a time when you have had to deal with a complaint against you or others.
* What management experience do you have?
* What is your strongest and weakest strength clinically?
* Tell me about a time when you used listening and non-verbal communication effectively.

During the interview you may be presented with a scenario that you will role-play with the interviewer. This acts as a test of how you cope under pressure and sees whether you can prioritise appropriately. Typically this scenario involves multiple difficulties occurring simultaneously. For example:

> *"It is 4.30pm and you are working in the laboratory finishing off a cytokine assay when you get called by the Gastroenterology FY1 doctor. An inpatient with known liver disease and oesophageal varices has arrived with haematemesis and is hypotensive and tachycardiac. The team registrar is on a night shift, and the two FY2 doctors are in protected teaching. The FY1 doctor also needs to leave in 20 minutes to catch a plane on holiday. You are the only Gastroenterology registrar contactable as the others are on a training day. How would you manage this situation?"*

Obviously this is a very challenging situation with the interviewer looking for the candidate to act in a confident, safe, professional and methodical manner, putting the patient safety first at all times.

Key points

- There is no escaping it – preparation is the key to success!
- Know your application form, know your research and publications
- Have a clear structure as to how you will respond to very common questions such as 'Why do you want this job?' – these should be gifts in the interview
- Be enthusiastic – you want to demonstrate to the interviewers how passionate you are to pursue an academic career
- Don't be surprised if interviewers probe your research – they want to see that you have insight into the limitations of your work and have an open mind to others' work
- Be clear on what an academic career involves – the good and the bad!
- Try and arrange a mock interview – it helps enormously, if only to give you experience of being under pressure before the real thing
- Stay calm, think before you speak – and go for it!

Success! What to do next?

Hooray! You not only survived the interview, you got the job. But what happens next? Typically just before the interview, you would have been asked to rank the posts available (if more than one) in order of your personal preference. All appointable candidates will also have been ranked so that the highest ranked candidate gets their first choice of post and so on. You will be issued an academic national training number (NTN (A)) and often will be required to register with the responsible academic institution and the trust in which you perform your clinical duties. You will need to agree start dates (which are usually fixed).

Next you need to make a number of decisions with your clinical and academic supervisors about how precisely to manage your ACF/CL.

Supervisors or academic training coordinators have often spent much time thinking about this and making plans since it is not easy to accommodate the academic time with clinical rotas etc. Discuss this urgently with your supervisor:

* ★ When can you start? How long do you expect to spend in this post?
* ★ How are you going to divide your time to accommodate your clinical and academic duties?
* ★ Are you going to take a block of academic time or a few days each week? Is this possible?
* ★ What are your ultimate aims of this post? (you should have had a strong sense of this before the interview).
* ★ Can you ensure your academic time coincides closely to when fellowship/ funding applications become available, e.g. if applying to do a PhD?
* ★ What is your area of interest and how is it best to gain exposure to this during your academic activities?

There is a lot to take in initially and often this plan will evolve and become clearer once you actually start. Make contact with the ACF/CL supervisor immediately and your training programme director so you can plan early.

■ Better luck next time... What happens next?

So it's not the result you wanted. The question is: what do you do next? In these circumstances it is hard not to feel disappointed, but all is not lost. Firstly, if you are unsuccessful in Round 1, watch out for Round 2, remembering that applying for an academic post does not stop you from applying for the mainstream clinical speciality training programmes. However, if you are determined to pursue an academic pathway, you still can but you have just learnt how to deal with rejection. Before re-applying, it may be worth considering the following:

* ★ Is this really what I want? Am I being realistic? If the answer to both is 'yes' then keep pursuing your dream.
* ★ Are there any areas that you can improve on in either the application or interview?
* ★ Speak to your supervisors, colleagues and other academics and ask their advice.
* ★ If there are gaps in your academic CV, work hard to fill them!
* ★ Believe in yourself – you can do it!

Academic qualifications

Higher degrees, diplomas and certificates

Luke Moore
Misha Moore
Beverley Almeida

Why do a higher degree, diploma or certificate?

In recent years postgraduate medical training has become more standardised. Most doctors graduate with degrees in medicine and surgery and some with an additional intercalated bachelor's degree. The majority then acquire their clinical qualifications – certification of completion of foundation training, membership of a Royal College, exit or speciality exams and certification of completion of training (CCT) with subsequent entry onto a specialist register. However changes to subspeciality training have again placed emphasis on open competitive allocation of posts, and competition for sought-after posts during this process is often strong. Furthermore, when you come to the end of this conveyor belt, how will you distinguish yourself at consultant interview and compete successfully for the post you really want? What will you offer an employer and colleagues over and above high-quality care of patients?

A doctorate (MD or PhD) has historically been a good way to distinguish yourself, but may be best done when your career plan is more developed and you have an idea of your professional goal. It is certainly crucial for those considering a full-time career in academic medicine. Higher degrees, diplomas and certificates can enable you to gain new skills, further your knowledge and broaden your experience earlier on in your professional careers. They not only allow you to develop as an individual and as a doctor but can also, and this should not be underestimated, develop your CV at any stage to make you stand out from those around you. For the majority of doctors who do not wish to pursue a PhD/MD then they also allow the acquisition of skills valuable to a consultant, specialist or GP principal.

> **Key points**
> - Consider carefully why you want to do the course
> - Will a diploma or certificate be sufficient for your purposes?
> - Research the course carefully – ask around and attend the university
> - Consider funding and geographical implications

In the highly competitive application rounds for core or more importantly, speciality training, pursuing such higher education may score valuable points in the application process. Even if points are not awarded specifically for higher degrees in the scoring system, they allow you to gain experiences and skills that can always be incorporated into several fields within the application form and interview to increase your chances of success. Whilst the need to score highly and obtain the training job of your choice is important, you must remember that this should never be the sole motivation, that pursuing higher education is a worthy end in itself and will provide you with invaluable skills. Indeed in some specialities such as public health a higher degree is mandatory and in some deaneries, a higher degree in certain specialities is also compulsory. Higher degrees, diplomas and certificates, if chosen correctly to suit you and your goals, are so much more than just stepping stones.

Choosing what to do

So what then do we mean by higher education? The hierarchies of qualification within this area can be confusing to the uninitiated. Here we concentrate on three common tiers of accreditation (doctorates are discussed in Chapter 8).

Postgraduate Certificate (PGCert)

These usually entail the least amount of work and consequently the specialised knowledge you obtain is less extensive than that from a diploma or a master's degree. Programmes are usually a collection of modules, some of which may be derived from those undertaken in the final year of complimentary undergraduate degrees. Studying for a certificate, if undertaken as a taught course, will usually entail over 100 hours of contact time, and as with all education, will require an additional two to four times this duration of private study. Depending on the nature of the programme, attainment of the certificate will be either through examination, continuous assessment or occasionally solely through essays and submitted projects. Some institutes state that attainment of a postgraduate certificate may be regarded as equivalent to honours in an undergraduate degree.

Postgraduate Diploma (PGDip or Dip)

Postgraduate diplomas are more involved than certificates, often requiring over 200 hours of contact time when undertaken as a taught course and may take up to 6 months if you choose to study the course full time. Assessment is usually by examination or by essay and occasionally by the completion of a project. Most institutes set the standard of a successful candidate as that of an undergraduate honours student or if for a vocational subject then success will be measured against the minimum standards set by the relevant professional body. Postgraduate diplomas can also be awarded to those who complete most or all of a master's degree programme but who choose not (or fail) to hand in their dissertation. In terms of credits, a postgraduate diploma usually represents 120 with a master's degree representing 180 credits.

Master's degree (MSc or MA or MBA)

In the UK, a 'higher degree' is any degree above a bachelor's, but the term is often used to mean a master's degree. In Europe however the phrase 'higher degree' often implies a degree *beyond* master's. The master's degree represents an academic award granted to candidates who have completed a programme of taught and independent study that may be in a specific area of knowledge or field of professional practice. Master's degrees usually facilitate not only acquisition of knowledge or skills by the candidate, but also practical application, critical evaluation and problem-solving skills in this area. Master's degrees are usually undertaken over the period of 1 year for a full-time student, or 2 years part time. Master's degrees studied by distance learning are often completed over a period of up to 5 years. Assessment is either through exams or assessed essays, but almost universally master's degrees include a dissertation project assessing the candidate's ability to undertake independent investigation.

Which to choose?

Clearly this will depend on what you are trying to achieve or gain, the nature of courses on offer and the time and funding available to you. Inevitably a master's degree is the most useful intellectually and in terms of career utility, but may not be available in the area of your choice, especially for more vocational subjects.

Choosing where to do it

The decision on where you do your higher education may be out of your hands. It will depend not only upon your geographical location, but also on the course you wish to undertake. Whilst geographically remote institutes can be considered for those wishing to study through distance learning (see later) those trying to intertwine part-time studies with work commitments will be limited to locally available courses. Some doctors wanting to undertake a specific higher education course through full-time study do move in order to do this, particularly for prestigious awards. You should consider this carefully however, as studying away from family and support mechanisms can make it significantly more difficult.

If you are lucky enough to have several institutes offering similar courses in your vicinity, then you will need to make an objective assessment of which course is best. This will involve assessment of the modules contained within the course programme and their relevance to you and your goals, assessment of the prestige of the institute, and often assessment of practical issues such as the exam structure and quantity of contact time. Cost may well be a factor in your decision and this varies enormously for home students (UK and EU) and those from overseas; full- versus part-time courses and also between institutions and universities. Take a look at the various ranking systems used to grade universities (such as www.rae.ac.uk) and check their websites for costs.

Funding higher education

The age-old problem of money can be a major factor in your decision to pursue a master's degree, diploma or certificate. As this activity is usually outside the remit of a standard Royal College curriculum this may have implications on your ability to take on higher education. Full-time courses will require a full year's tuition fees at the start of the course, whereas part-time courses will be paid over the 2 (or more) years over which you complete your study. This may mean proportionally you pay more as tuition fees tend to rise each year. Alternatively this allows you to spread the cost of your course and for some degrees completed in a modular manner this again may soften the blow. However, exactly what you're charged depends on the university with which you enrol, your course, where in the UK you study and whether you are classified as a home or overseas student. This latter distinction is crucial, can vary by university (though should not) and can make thousands of pounds difference in the cost of a course. You must ask carefully about this at the university. Hopefully financing your master's degree, diploma or certificate will not be the sole stumbling block.

Funding for research-based projects as part of MDs or PhD is discussed in detail in Chapter 9, but some brief ideas for funding of courses are outlined here.

Grants, educational trusts and local hospital trust funds

These are all potential options for obtaining money to support you financially. Some educational trusts specifically support individuals pursuing higher education and provide grants for this purpose. In addition, your local hospital may have trust funds that can be accessed for higher education if you complete your dissertation in an area that could benefit both parties. Your local medical library will have lists of such contacts, or the local university.

Study leave budgets

A proportion of your study leave budget may be utilised towards your course fees. This is however not uniformly true across the UK, and depends on the deanery, hospital trust and director of medical education. Using your study leave budget may have an impact on other courses that may be mandatory as part of your Royal College curriculum, but a proportion could be set aside to help. Those individuals whose deanery dictates a master's degree is compulsory may have their entire study leave budget offset against the course fees, so the decision to use study leave funds will have already been made. Even if you are unable to use any of your study leave budget (if you have one) you will still need to apply for study leave (time) in order to attend your course, and you must consider whether this is permitted within your rota and your commitment to service provision.

Self-funding

This is how most junior doctors fund their further study. You are lucky if you are in a position to be able to do this, but you must take into account your other financial commitments and whether this is personally feasible. For example, undertaking extra locum work at weekends may generate income but may not leave you time actually to study and may affect your performance at work.

Fitting it all in

There are several ways for you practically to go about studying for a higher award, but fitting these studies in and around your clinical commitments may present a challenge. Before you even think about undertaking higher education, you need to think about the approach you are going to take. There are three main avenues to consider:

Full time

Programme durations for certificates and diplomas vary and are not necessarily in line with the academic kudos of the award – for example a full-time Postgraduate Certificate in Education usually takes at least two if not three terms (almost 1 year), whilst the Diploma of Tropical Medicine and Hygiene takes 3 months. Master's degrees in the UK take 1 year in most instances. You can see that whilst your study leave entitlement as a practicing doctor is great for short courses, it just isn't compatible with a full-time higher award. You therefore only have one real option if you wish to complete one of these programmes full time – take some time out from clinical training.

You may feel you are in a position to do this between completing your foundation years and taking up your core or speciality training. Indeed for those core or speciality training posts with an August changeover, this fits well with the academic year, especially for year-long courses such as master's degrees. You would then be able to apply for core/speciality posts the following year. This can be even more convenient if your core or speciality training starts in September or October. However be aware that this is a period when you have just acquired your core foundation clinical skills and people may have reservations about this being the best time to take a complete break from clinical work. If you do take a higher degree at this stage that lasts for less than 1 academic year then you may wish also to obtain structured clinical experience or even overseas experience for the remainder of the time available to you. Be aware that taking 1 year out between F1 and F2 years is not possible nor between CT1 and CT2 years in core medicine or core surgery training, without some very exceptional reason. If you are taking time out during other training programmes (e.g. paediatrics, higher medical or surgical training, psychiatry, etc.) you must formally apply for the time as an 'out-of-programme experience' (OOPE) or 'out-of-programme for research' (OOPR) from your deanery and training programme director. Whilst OOPEs should be relevant to your training, even distant subjects may be approved if you can make a strong case for how they would enhance your skills and be relevant to your future career. There are a standard set of forms that must be completed (available from your deanery) and countersigned by your training programme director and educational supervisor, and a minimum of 6 months' notice is required. Some training programmes will only be able to release you at fixed points in the year to ensure minimal gaps in programmes, detrimental effects on patient care and other trainees.

Key points

- All OOP periods (experience, research, career breaks or training) require formal paperwork to be completed in a timely fashion with your deanery
- OOPE and OOPR is a privilege and not an automatic right, approach your deanery and your Specialist Training Committee (STC) chair or training programme director to discuss your plans
- Don't miss the deanery deadlines otherwise you may need to drop out of your course
- Plan at least a year ahead of time

You should be deterred from lazing about until you apply for your next job – such gaps on your CV are difficult to explain at interview! If you are unsuccessful in obtaining a training number, a higher degree may provide a more honourable entry on your CV compared to a career gap.

You should bear in mind however that the Gold Guide (the formal framework covering all training programmes in the UK) suggests that only 3 years of OOP allowance can be given to any one trainee. Therefore care needs to be taken in planning your OOPE if you may consider doing a 3-year doctorate or 2-year MD at a later point. Discuss this at an early stage with your training programme director. Most deaneries would not prevent you undertaking a competitively won research training fellowship for 3 years even if you had already done a 1-year MSc, but this is not an automatic entitlement. Don't forget to think of the effects of time out on your overall life plan if this is relevant. Your CCT date will be delayed. Taking more than 3 months completely out of the NHS can result in loss of maternity pay entitlements on your return. There may be important consequences if you were to get pregnant during a gap or even immediately on your return to clinical training. Some people may also consider the effects of loss of NHS income for the time period on your subsequent NHS pension. Speak to your human resources department if this might affect you.

Part time

One alternative to pursuing a full-time higher award is to attempt to do it part time. Choosing to undertake a programme in this way will limit the number of courses available to you since only certain institutes and certain disciplines provide this mode of study. If the higher award is mandatory for your speciality, posts may be organised to incorporate certain days off a week to cater for this. If not, this route can be difficult as ensuring you get the same days off every week (for example) as part of study leave is likely to be at odds with clinical commitments and service provision and may be impossible in practice.

Some courses are easier to blend into your clinical commitments than others and you should always liaise closely with your educational supervisor, your clinical supervisor, training programme director and rota coordinators before committing yourself. The other practical aspect that does need to be considered is that many clinical rotations, whether at foundation or speciality level, cycle trainees through various different trusts or GP practices. Therefore if you are contemplating part-time study, and the timeframe does cross a job changeover, make sure you discuss it with *both* trusts/employers. It may be that a suitable option is to discuss your plans with the deanery to make a case for applying to work as a less than full-time trainee. The financial considerations of this, as well as the effect of delaying your CCT date should be borne in mind. Flexible (less than full time) work is also increasingly difficult to obtain since this requires supernumerary funding from the deanery, which is increasingly restricted unless you can arrange a job share with a colleague.

Endurance is a key personal attribute since part-time courses take longer to complete than full time, with a part-time master's degree typically taking 2 years. Part-time study may involve less contact time and is spread over a longer period. As such self-motivation and self-discipline are vital when it comes to finding time to knuckle down to study.

Distance learning

The last main avenue you may wish to consider in pursuing higher education is that of distance learning. For a busy doctor with immobile clinical commitments this may ostensibly appear to be the perfect option – minimal contact time, with learning achieved through modules you work through in your own time (either posted to you or online), and assessment through essays submitted from a distance, and exams as necessary on a few days at the end of the course. Many institutes offer certificates, diplomas and degrees via this method, and in a wide range of disciplines. Distance learning is often set up in a modular fashion, and can be undertaken a few modules at a time often over a prolonged period. Most distance master's degrees for example can be completed over 2–5 years. However many subjects, particularly the more practical ones, are not generally available through distance learning.

You certainly need to be determined, disciplined and able to show endurance to undertake part-time education. This is multiplied 100-fold when pursuing distance learning – you will have minimal direct contact time with teachers, and you will be in complete charge of timing your progress through the modules in order to meet the apparently distant essay and exam assessments. This may seem easy at first glance, but you need to factor in your on-call periods, the presentations you'll have to give at work, the papers you'll have to write for your professor, local audits, the conferences you'll be going to, clinical training days etc. It all soon mounts up. Whilst distance learning is the ultimate answer for some, it is quite the ultimate disaster for others.

▣ Master's degrees, diplomas, certificates – is there one for you?

The following section outlines specific examples of higher education most suitable for clinicians with a medical degree as their undergraduate degree. There is brief guidance as to how the course is taught, how assessments take place and which universities provide them. This is an extensive but not exhaustive list and hopefully will give you an idea of what you might like to apply for and help focus your thoughts. Bear in mind that new courses are always becoming available (and old ones closing) and given the constraints of junior doctors' rotas the manner in which they are delivered is constantly changing. Therefore consider this list as an outline and something to stimulate ideas; it should not be a substitute for picking up a university prospectus or doing your own online search.

Generic

Clinical Trials, Health Research, Clinical Research

* **Available levels:** MSc, PGDip, PGCert.
* **Available from:** London School of Hygiene & Tropical Medicine, University of Leeds, University of Durham, University of Cardiff, University of Sheffield, University of Cranfield, University of Leeds.

* **Available through:** Full time, part time, distance learning.
* **Why do it?:** You may want a thorough grounding in research methods perhaps to aid research in your clinical career or to further an academic career. These courses furnish a range of techniques and skills required to undertake high-quality clinical research.
* **What it involves:** Core modules will include fundamentals of research methodology and statistics. Examples of advanced modules include ethics, economic evaluation, epidemiology and data analysis. A dissertation is generally required.
* **Is it worth it?:** These courses provide an excellent grounding in the research methodology that we rarely obtain during our undergraduate education. Whilst some find this advantageous, especially if they are carving out an academic career, others may be happier to learn 'on the job' if they are hoping to carry out an MD as part of a predominantly clinical career. This qualification may support doctors wishing to participate in trial design, oversight and management for pharmaceutical companies, the NHS or other research organisations.

Healthcare Ethics/Medical Law

* **Available levels:** MSc, MA, LLM (master's in law), PGDip, PGCert.
* **Available from:** *Ethics* Univeristy of Leeds. *Law* University of Cardiff, University of Glasgow, University of Northumbria. *Combined* University of Bristol, University of Manchester, University of Dundee, University of Liverpool, University of Edinburgh, University of Kent, King's College London, Queen Mary (University of London), De Montfort University.
* **Available through:** Full time, part time, distance learning (Dundee, Edinburgh, De Montfort).
* **Why do it?:** A range of courses are offered in various institutions incorporating medical law and ethics either singly or in combination. These courses are designed to attract those interested in the legal aspects of clinical practice that are tightly linked to medical ethics. This may help in developing a more rounded approach to your own clinical practice and enabling a more holistic approach to medicine. It may also be useful for those aspiring to roles in management, or provide a base for further academic work. It could even be useful for those who end up with subsidiary interests further along the career pathway such as those who take up the role of expert witnesses or other medico–legal work. Ethical and legal principles are also useful for those who might want to be involved with clinical research, trial design, ethics committees, clinical management and clinical teaching.
* **What it involves:** Courses vary but generally involve core modules laying the foundations of ethics and legal aspects of medicine, followed by optional modules and often a dissertation. Assessment takes the form of either written assignments, exams or both.

★ **Is it worth it?:** Medical ethics gets bad press as a 'wishy washy' subject, but don't underestimate how often you will subliminally use its principles in your clinical work, teaching and even research. With the growing importance of ethical issues and litigation in medicine a deeper understanding of these subjects can only be useful. Be sure you know what you aim to gain – a master's in law will not enable you to practice medical law, which requires law conversion followed by further training.

Medical Education and Surgical Education

★ **Available levels:** MMedEd/MSurgEd, PGDip, PGCert.
★ **Available from:** University College London (in conjunction with the RCP), University of Warwick, University of Bedfordshire, University of Nottingham, University of Cardiff, University of Dundee, Imperial College London (MSurgEd).
★ **Available through:** Full time, part time, distance learning.
★ **Why do it?:** These are often undertaken by those who would like to take on educational leadership roles or incorporate education and training into their clinical practice. It allows you to explore the theoretical side of education and learning and to develop your knowledge of teaching methods, appraisal, evaluation and research skills. Such courses are also integrated into some fellowships in medical education, which can be taken as OOPE.
★ **What it involves:** Courses vary in their content but almost all include compulsory modules in educational theory. Other modules may include teaching methods, research methodology, informatics, appraisal, evaluation and clinical simulation. Assessment ranges from essays, projects, dissertations and practical assignments (including observed teaching) depending on the institution.
★ **Is it worth it?:** It is becoming increasingly recognised that medical education requires a structured approach and that trainers and teachers should be suitably qualified. A master's in medical and surgical education will provide evidence of this if you choose to take up an educational leadership role in the future. Increasingly you will require some formal evidence of training in teaching/training or a higher qualification if you want this to be a major feature of your work.

Medical Leadership and Clinical Leadership

★ **Available levels:** MSc, PGDip, PGCert.
★ **Available from:** Royal College of Physicians of London, University of Glasgow, University of Warwick.
★ **Available through:** Part time learning only.
★ **Why do it?:** This qualification is really aimed at those who have a desire to enter hospital higher management structures. As doctors, we are all both managed by others and manage those under our supervision, and increasingly clinicians provide the mainstay of hospital management and

leadership. Pursuing higher education in Medical or Clinical Leadership will develop your knowledge of organisational behaviour, good practice, occupational psychology and you own personal leadership qualities, all with the aim of aiding you to become better clinical leaders.

* **What it involves:** The RCP London course involves 14 contact days in the first year (PGCert), 13 contact days in the second year (PGDip) and a supervised research project (MSc) that can either be completed during these 2 years or the following year. Assessment is through written coursework, presentations and group work during the contact days.
* **Is it worth it?:** This provides knowledge and understanding to develop you into an effective leader in your field and if you pick your institution can allow you to become acquainted with some very influential peers.

Public Health: MPH

* **Available levels:** MSc, PGDip, PGCert.
* **Available from:** Several universities including: London School of Hygiene and Tropical Medicine, University of Liverpool, Imperial College London, University of Glasgow, University of Manchester, University of Leeds, King's College London, University of Sheffield, University of Nottingham, University of Edinburgh, University of Dundee, University of Birmingham.
* **Available through:** Full time, part time, distance learning.
* **Why do it?:** A master's in public health is compulsory for those on the public health training scheme and is generally funded. It can be useful for anyone interested in public health or those who might consider taking on related managerial or political roles in the future. In some countries outside the UK it is possible to become a public health specialist after obtaining an MPH without necessarily having completed a training scheme.
* **What it involves:** Compulsory modules (e.g. epidemiology, statistics, health economics etc.) lay the theoretical foundations of public health. This is followed by optional modules and generally a dissertation or project. Assessment may be via written assignments, assessed group work, assessed presentations and exams.
* **Is it worth it?:** The MPH generally gets good feedback. Graduates find they have a wider appreciation of healthcare and gain transferable skills such as those in statistics, epidemiology and research methodology. If you are on the public health training scheme it is compulsory for your training. If you feel you want to develop your knowledge in one related area, certain institutions provide master's in subjects such as epidemiology or statistics in isolation.

General practice

Clinical Dermatology

* **Available levels:** MSc, PGDip.

* **Available from:** Kings College London, University of Cardiff, Queen Mary University London.
* **Available through:** Full time, part time (PGdip QMUL).
* **Why do it?:** You may want to specialise in dermatology after your general medical training or be a GP with a special interest in dermatology. These courses provide a firm scientific grounding in dermatology. They also have a clinical emphasis with a substantial practical component.
* **What it involves:** The courses utilise didactic teaching, clinical sessions and laboratory sessions. Assessment is through examinations, written assignments and a research project or dissertation.
* **Is it worth it?:** A higher qualification in clinical dermatology can provide a useful adjunct to specialist training programmes. For GPs, dermatology is a frequently seen but poorly taught subject. The MSc could help you pursue it as a special interest, which may also assist in securing hospital sessions with financial incentives attached.

Primary Care or General Practice

* **Available levels:** MSc, PGDip, PGCert.
* **Available from:** King's College London, City University, University of Ulster, University of Leeds, University of Birmingham, University of Central Lancashire, Institute of Health Science Education (Bart's and the London).
* **Available through:** Full time, part time, distance learning.
* **Why do it?:** These courses aim to provide in-depth knowledge of academic, clinical and management issues in primary care and are often aimed at other members of the primary care team as well as general practitioners.
* **What it involves:** Courses vary depending on the institution, however, may include modules on evidence-based clinical practice, health service delivery, research methods and management. Assessment is often through written assignments, although exams and dissertations may also be used.
* **Is it worth it?:** This will depend on personal opinion. Some working in primary care may not see the clinical relevance of a master's. Those who are interested in leadership roles, policy making, research or even development of primary care abroad will find these courses rewarding. Academic general practice is a fast-developing subspeciality and a part- or full-time post in a university department of general practice will require a higher degree. Furthermore, such higher degrees can help you gain positions on central general practice organisations or committees.

Sports Medicine

* **Available levels:** MSc, PGDip.
* **Available from:** University College London, University of Bath, University of Nottingham, University of Exeter, University of Glasgow, Queen Mary University London.
* **Available through:** Full time, part time, distance learning.

* **Why do it?:** These courses are aimed at those considering a career in sports medicine. They may be relevant for GPs with special interests in the field, rheumatologists or orthopaedic surgeons, or alternatively could act as a brownie point towards getting into sports and exercise medicine speciality training.
* **What it involves:** Most courses (apart from distance learning) incorporate both theoretical and practical components. These include lectures, field trips, clinics and other practical sessions. Assessment is via coursework and exams and may include a dissertation.
* **Is it worth it?:** A sports medicine diploma is not a prerequisite for entry into the speciality training programme, however, many applicants will have one and that will increase their chances of success (although this is not a very competitive speciality). Doing the course demonstrates your commitment and should allow you to give better examples of your knowledge on an application form and at interviews. For GPs sports medicine can be practiced as a special interest, often with attractive financial incentives, and it is difficult to gain substantial training in the subject simply through the GP training programmes.

Medicine

Cardiology

* **Available levels:** MSc, PGDip, PGCert.
* **Available from:** Imperial College London (MSc in Preventative Cardiology), University of Brighton and Canterbury Christ Church University.
* **Available through:** Full time or part time.
* **Why do it?:** Cardiology remains a competitive speciality and your ward-based exposure during core medical training may not be sufficient to gain a training number. While not only demonstrating your commitment, these courses will cover key knowledge helpful for your early years in subspeciality training.
* **What it involves:** The Imperial MSc (also offered as a certificate of advanced study) has a specific focus on preventative strategies such as cholesterol and hypertension control. It is delivered by a multidisciplinary team of course organisers including dieticians, physiotherapists and pharmacists. As such, course attendees are from a varied background. The course is divided into modules of didactic learning, tutorials and practical clinical visits. The MSc courses at Canterbury (taught at the Medway campus) and at the University of Brighton are more general with the option of modules including acute cardiology, research methods and education. All three MSc courses require a dissertation.
* **Is it really worth it?:** In general you may do this to boost your CV at core training level, although it is not clear whether this is especially useful. In the past, cardiology trainees had to have a doctorate (MD or PhD) to get a training number. Now it is more typical for trainees to do doctorate research as an OOPR during training. An MSc may help support your progress from

CT2 in Medicine to ST3 in Cardiology. However, you may wish to undertake an MD or PhD earlier to avoid doing it when you are ready to choose your cardiology subspeciality. The Preventive Cardiology MSc will be helpful if you wish to pursue that subspeciality in the future, but again consider it a base from which to support an MD to gain a consultant post.

Endocrinology and Diabetes

* **Available levels:** MSc, PGDip, PGCert.
* **Available from:** Universities of Warwick, Leicester, Edinburgh, Brighton, Queen Mary University of London and Kings College London.
* **Available through:** Full time or part time.
* **Why do it?:** Several of the above-mentioned courses are designed specifically with speciality trainees in mind, aiming to cover all the areas of clinical endocrinology required for speciality certificate exams. The course offered by Kings also offers a particularly well-regarded module on research design, statistics, ethics and methodology that prepares candidates well not only for the research-based dissertation those studying at MSc level must complete, but also may prepare them for future research.
* **What is involved:** The usual mix of in-course assessments and exams and dissertation for the MSc. For the Kings course those not in a London deanery training post will have to be interviewed prior to acceptance on the course.
* **Is it really worth it?:** Provides a good grounding in an often complicated subject and if you pursue the right line of study can prepare your research skills well for future projects in this field.

Gastroenterology

* **Available levels:** MSc, PGDip, PGCert.
* **Available from:** The best known is that offered by the Centre for Gastroenterology through Queen Mary University of London, although there is an MSc available to North West STC trainees offered by the University of Salford.
* **Available through:** Full time or part time.
* **Why do it?:** Not only is the curriculum of this course designed to cover the three subspecialties of gastroenterology, hepatology and nutrition in detail, but a very practically orientated module on endoscopy allows you to understand the principles of how to run an endoscopy service as well as develop core skills using endoscopy simulators.
* **What it involves:** Taught modules run between October and April and are assessed by modular coursework and compulsory exams. For those pursuing this at MSc level, a dissertation must be submitted.
* **Is it really worth it?:** This course may provide a base from which you can develop your own learning while training in gastroenterology. The endoscopy component is good, but is no replacement for routine clinical endoscopy lists and the JAG (Joint Advisory Group on GI endoscopy) courses.

Geriatric Medicine and Gerontology

★ **Available levels:** MSc, PGDip (including the DGM), PGCert.
★ **Available from:** Kings College London, Universities of Southampton, Cardiff, Salford, Keele and Brighton (the Royal College of Physicians of London offer the Diploma of Geriatric Medicine only).
★ **Available through:** Full time or part time.
★ **Why do it?:** Both physicians with a special interest in gerontology and GPs can develop their knowledge and understanding of older people from biological, psychosocial, and demographic perspectives and also develop wider ranging insights into related government policy, health service structure and societal perspectives. The Diploma in Geriatric Medicine (DGM) from the Royal College of Physicians of London is a specific vocational qualification particularly aimed at general practice trainees and those working in non-consultant career posts in departments of geriatric medicine.
★ **What it involves:** Most of the institutions offering these courses require 1 day per week contact for part-time students and 2 days per week for full-time students with different modules assessed through essays and/or exams. Those aiming for a master's degree will have to undertake a supervised research-based dissertation.
★ **Is it worth it?:** Those studying on these courses are often from varied professional backgrounds, which creates a beneficial learning environment. The teaching on the wider aspects of gerontology provides invaluable preparation for consultant posts in geriatric medicine, and the dissertation project can provide experience of clinical research in this field that you can take forward in your future career.

Infectious Diseases, Clinical Microbiology, Tropical Medicine, Medical Mycology and Medical Parasitology

★ **Available levels:** MSc, PGDip (including DTM&H), PGCert.
★ **Available from:** London School of Hygiene and Tropical Medicine (LSHTM), Liverpool School of Tropical Medicine (LSTM), Queen Mary University of London, University College London, Universities of Nottingham and Edinburgh.
★ **Available through:** Full time or part time, some courses through distance learning.
★ **Why do it?:** The field of infection has always been one of the more academically orientated medical specialties and competition for training in this field is fierce. Some of the qualifications mentioned above are often undertaken through distance learning by those aiming to secure a training number (such as the MSc in Infectious Diseases) whilst others are studied by those already in training posts who are trying to develop a special interest in one subspeciality (such as mycology or parasitology) who often undertake part-time courses. The Diploma of Tropical Medicine & Hygiene (DTM&H)

is a particular qualification offered by LSHTM and LSTM on a full-time basis lasting 3 months and covers all aspects of practicing tropical medicine. It has a particularly practical approach and is often undertaken by those aiming to practice or research in tropical areas.

* **What it involves:** Most of these courses blend lectures with laboratory practicals. The lectures vary from clinical aspects of infection through diagnostic approaches to wider ranging public health issues and strategies for communicable disease control. Each course will have different blends of learning and you should investigate which course will meet your individual education needs and career goals. Assessment for these qualifications can be arduous, with the majority of these courses having synoptic exams.
* **Is it really worth it?:** Proving your commitment to the field of infection can make all the difference in advancing your career in this field and pursuing higher qualifications is certainly one way to do this. Many courses also provide firm groundings in statistics and epidemiology that can prove exceptionally useful for future research projects. If you are trying to pursue an infectious diseases career you should discuss all your options thoroughly with those already in posts as clinical experience of infectious diseases and often tropical experience can be key.

Diploma in the Medical Care of Catastrophes

* **Available from:** Worshipful Society of Apothecaries.
* **Available through:** Part-time study only.
* **Why do it?:** This course is designed as very real preparation for those aiming to work in catastrophe situations and aims to establish a cross-speciality level of skill.
* **What it involves:** The course occurs on 12 Saturdays spread over a calendar year, culminating in a written and OSCE exam with a dissertation submission.
* **Is it worth it?:** For those aiming to work in the Tropics, most would advocate taking either the DTM&H or the DMCC – and if you are a career low-resource setting doctor, perhaps both!

Nephrology

* **Available levels:** MSc, PGDip, PGCert.
* **Available from:** University of Brighton, Sheffield Kidney Institute (also offers PGDip).
* **Available through:** Full time or part time.
* **Why do it?:** This degree is open to a range of renal medicine practitioners but is billed as being ideal for first and second year speciality registrars in nephrology. The syllabus covers everything from pathophysiology to disease management and is very clinically orientated. The course offered through Brighton also allows you to bring in additional education or management modules if you are interested in broadening the scope of your learning.

* **What it involves:** Brighton: Each of the modules is concentrated into a 5-day week, which may make part-time study easier for some. For those undertaking this mode of study it is suggested you take three modules each year for 2 years with the dissertation being planned in the second and written in the third year. It is strongly suggested that you have employment within a unit in which you are involved in day-to-day care of renal patients, and there is an interview prior to acceptance onto the course. The Sheffield MSc is full time and includes modules on all aspects of nephrology including transplantation, tropical nephrology, statistics etc.
* **Is it worth it?:** This qualification can be both brownie points on your CV, especially if you are not undertaking a PhD/MD and meet your learning needs for the Speciality Certificate Examination.

Palliative Medicine

* **Available levels:** MSc, PGDip, PGCert.
* **Available from:** University of Cardiff, University of Bristol, Kings College London.
* **Available through:** Full time, part time or distance learning.
* **Why do it?:** These courses add structure to your learning in this field and cover most of the curriculum likely to be examined when Specialty Certificate Examinations begin in palliative care in 2011.
* **What it involves:** Distance-learning modules can be undertaken at your own rate; the Cardiff course does require some residential weekends. The dissertation at MSc level will require some novel research and you should ensure you have a mechanism in place to be able to do this.
* **Is it worth it?:** If you are just looking for a structure to your learning, the diploma level should be sufficient, but pursuing the MSc will give you the opportunity to develop your research ability and you may be able to publish your work, further boosting your CV.

Sexually Transmitted Infections and Human Immunodeficiency Virus, and Genitourinary Medicine

* **Available levels:** MSc, PGDip (including Dip GUM and Dip HIV Medicine), PGCert.
* **Available from:** LSHTM and University College London (Dip GUM and Dip HIV Medicine run by the Worshipful Society of Apothecaries (WSA) of London).
* **Available through:** Full time or part time.
* **Why do it?:** Learning ranges from the laboratory aspects of these diseases including practical microscopy to the pathophysiology, epidemiology, clinical management and wider public health issues. The WSA offers two diplomas in this field – the Dip GUM is *compulsory* for speciality trainees in genitourinary medicine and whilst the Dip HIV Medicine is not; it is still a sought-after qualification.

* **What it involves:** Core and advanced modules in the various areas of STI and HIV medicine with the dissertation for those taking this at master's level often being undertaken in a relevant overseas location. The Dip GUM examination is supported by WSA and BASHH courses.
* **Is it worth it?:** Other than the fact that the Dip GUM is compulsory, the other courses are very up to date in a field that is full of fast-moving developments.

Diploma of Travel Medicine

* **Available from:** Royal College of Physicians and Surgeons (Glasgow).
* **Available through:** Blended part time and distance learning only.
* **Why do it?:** This course aims to develop theoretical and practically orientated knowledge in those practising preventative medicine for travellers. It is a qualification sought after by both NHS and private travel clinics.
* **What it involves:** Taught over a calendar year, the course involves two 1-week residential courses in Glasgow and distance-learning modules covering a variety of travel disease and disease prevention topics culminating in written and practical exams.
* **Is it worth it?:** This course is great for those specialising in this field and also for generalists who may have an interest or a clinical need to further their knowledge in travel medicine.

Surgery

Colorectal Surgery and Colonoscopy

* **Available levels:** MSc, PGDip, PGCert.
* **Available from:** University of Hull.
* **Available through:** Full time or part time/distance learning blended study.
* **Why do it?:** The colonoscopy course covers not only the theory and practice of colonoscopy but also critical thinking and research skills. The colorectal surgery course is practically orientated and aims to provide a structured approach to developing your knowledge and skills in this area.
* **What it involves:** The majority of the teaching through distance learning is delivered online, supplemented by study days that underpin the theory components. Those intending to study colonoscopy must be eligible for Joint Advisory Group on GI endoscopy (JAG) registration.
* **Is it worth it?:** Think carefully about your ability to pursue either of these courses and how much they will benefit you. They may provide opportunities for skill development you cannot gain elsewhere and a worthwhile accreditation but depending upon your educational needs you may be able to find alternatives. They will not make up for the need for practical experience and training in JAG-accredited training centres.

Diploma in Aesthetic Surgery

* **Available levels:** PGDip.
* **Available from:** Queen Mary University of London.

* **Available through:** Distance learning only.
* **Why do it?:** Training in aesthetic aspects of plastic surgery in the UK NHS system can present a challenge. This diploma is structured to cover the practical aspects of this field and this is well supported by specific 'contact' days via live video links with Q&A sessions into theatre.
* **What it involves:** The course material is comprehensive and comes as papers and DVDs. There is a weekly commitment to return assignments and you must attend the 'contact' days. Assessment is through written and viva examinations.
* **Is it worth it?:** The course is ideal for those training in plastic surgery who wish to develop a special interest in aesthetics, but should ideally be undertaken by those who are able to consolidate the learning from this course through further clinical practice. Beware this course is not cheap.

Oral and Maxillo-facial and Ear Nose and Throat

* **Available levels:** MSc and the Diploma of Head & Neck Surgery (DOHNS).
* **Available from:** Universities of Manchester, Sheffield, Glasgow and University College London (DOHNS from the Royal College of Surgeons).
* **Available through:** Full time or part time.
* **Why do it?:** These courses cover not only the pathophysiology of oral and maxillo-facial disease and current investigation and management, but also cover theory and laboratory practice of oro-facial technology. Several of the courses listed earlier are particularly clinically orientated, requiring participation in clinics and allowing observation of theatre sessions. The diploma in otolaryngology/head and neck surgery is an intercollegiate qualification aimed at those wishing to practice otolaryngology at a non-consultant grade.
* **What it involves:** These MSc courses can be contact-time intensive and are particularly expensive for a master's degree so consider carefully before committing yourself. The DOHNS is a vocational diploma examination consisting of written and OSCE assessments.
* **Is it worth it?:** The MSc courses offer unequalled experience and are a great way to boost your CV, however timing this course to fit in with your training will be difficult and you should work with your consultants to see how you might be able to accomplish this.

Surgical Science

* **Available levels:** MSc, PGDip, PGCert.
* **Available from:** Universities of Hull, Cardiff, Birmingham, Edinburgh, Queen Mary University of London and Imperial College London.
* **Available through:** Full time, part time or distance learning.
* **Why do it?:** These courses are well suited to trainee surgeons and teach both basic sciences and research methodology. In addition they often provide the opportunity to acquire experience in your chosen speciality and at MSc level allow you to develop and complete a piece of clinical or applied research.

* **What it involves:** As you will have read earlier, studying outside of your clinical work is not easy, so many who undertake part-time study take these courses close to their place of work. Perhaps the most flexible of the above institutions offering this course is Edinburgh, which operates through an online learning environment within course and end-of-year assessments.
* **Is it worth it?:** For many the prospect of trying to get a training number in surgery is a daunting task but this qualification can be pursued at or before core level and will not only give you something to discuss at interview but you may be able to publish your dissertation if it is of a high standard. The research methodology modules will also better prepare those aiming to complete doctorates in the future.

Trauma and Orthopaedics

* **Available levels:** MSc, PGDip (including Diploma in Hand Surgery), PGCert.
* **Available from:** Universities of Teeside, Salford, Warwick and Swansea, University College London. DHS from University of Manchester.
* **Available through:** Full time, part time or distance learning.
* **Why do it?:** These courses are ideal preparation for the FRCS(Orth) exam and can also provide opportunities to advance your understanding of paediatric and oncological orthopaedic problems. The Diploma of Hand Surgery (DHS) is aimed at new consultants and senior speciality trainees who wish to develop expertise in hand surgery.
* **What it involves:** The DHS is usually studied over 9–12 months but can be studied over a period of up to 24 months and must be undertaken whilst you are being supervised by a consultant who can assist you with practical experience.
* **Is it worth it?:** The Trauma and Orthopaedics (T&O) courses can definitely help to set you ahead of your colleagues in the current competitive market. There are several different institutes that offer these courses so pick the one that will extend your previous experiences. For those set on hand surgery, the DHS is a must.

Urology

* **Available levels:** MSc, PGDip.
* **Available from:** University College London.
* **Available through:** Part time only.
* **Why do it?:** This is a good way to develop a better understanding of the scientific basis of urology and particularly the importance of laboratory research and how to apply these methods.
* **What it involves:** Attendance at UCL for each of 10 Fridays per term over 2–4 years with multiple-choice question (MCQ) and viva exams, and for the MSc a research-based dissertation.

* **Is it worth it?:** This course is well suited to those aiming to undertake a research degree at a later stage, and the statistics and research methodology teaching will stand you in good stead. Going for MSc level is strongly advised – the research project, whilst onerous, may be developed into a publishable article if of sufficient quality.

Anaesthesia

Anaesthetics Research and Evidence-based Medicine Anaesthesia

* **Available levels:** MSc.
* **Available from:** University of Oxford and University of Teeside.
* **Available through:** Full time, part time or distance learning.
* **Why do it?:** These two postgraduate degree courses are aimed at speciality trainees in the field of anaesthesia. The Oxford-based anaesthesia research course would be ideally suited to those developing their research interest but do not yet wish to undertake a doctorate. The scope of research interests catered for at Oxford is very broad and the quality of the research is difficult to rival. The Teeside part-time degree in evidence-based medicine (EBM) anaesthesia is aimed at post fellowship speciality trainees and not only consolidates core knowledge but will importantly develop your research techniques in preparation for the MSc dissertation and for future projects.
* **What it involves:** The Teeside degree is particularly flexible but care must be taken in choosing your research project if you are undertaking this course as distance learning – as supervision can be tricky. Before considering the Oxford degree, think carefully about your research interests and discuss these in detail with the course organiser.
* **Is it really worth it?:** Whilst useful qualifications in their own right, both degrees can be good stepping stones to a doctorate.

Critical Care

* **Available levels:** MSc, PGDip (including Diploma in Intensive Care Medicine and European Diploma in Intensive Care), PGCert.
* **Available from:** University of Cardiff (DICM from Intercollegiate Board for Training in Intensive Care Medicine and EDIC from European Society of Intensive Care Medicine).
* **Available through:** Distance learning only.
* **Why do it?:** Pursuing one of these two qualifications provides structure to your learning in the field of intensive care, and will develop your ability to critically appraise information in a field that can move rapidly.
* **What it involves:** Make no mistake about these being easy qualifications. The course from Cardiff has been previously undertaken by those in their SHO years, but the entry criteria for the DCIM and EDIC are strict, and once eligible, the exams can be daunting, particularly the vivas. The dissertations can take a hefty amount of time so be prepared and balance this against any other professional exams you may need to study for.

* **Is it worth it?:** Undertaking the Cardiff course will develop your basic level of understanding in all areas of critical care, whilst the two more clinically orientated diplomas will develop your decision making and practical ability markedly. The DICM is particularly well respected in the UK.

Diploma of Anaesthesia, Trauma and Critical Care

* **Available from:** Accredited by the Royal College of Anaesthetists.
* **Available through:** Short course attendance then distance dissertation.
* **Why do it?:** This practically orientated diploma is aimed at those involved in the pre-hospital and resuscitation room management of patients with multiple trauma.
* **What it involves:** This diploma is no easy ride. You will need to score highly at the 3-day ATACC course (with assessment via a written and practical exam) before being accepted as a diploma candidate. You must then submit a substantial dissertation and meet several professional criteria.
* **Is it worth it?:** For those with an interest in pre-hospital management and resuscitation of poly-trauma victims this diploma is highly recommended for developing your clinical ability.

Pain Management

* **Available levels**: MSc, PGDip, PGCert.
* **Available from:** Universities of Leicester, Cardiff, Birmingham, Keele, Edinburgh and Queens Belfast.
* **Available through:** Full time, part time or distance learning.
* **Why do it?:** Courses in this area are particularly clinically orientated, covering relevant basic sciences and pain concepts and then focusing on clinical approaches and procedures in both acute and chronic pain management.
* **What it involves:** The breadth of universities offering this degree means that you should be able to find a learning style suitable for you. Read the prospectuses and think about how you can get the most out of each course.
* **Is it worth it?:** These courses are popular for a reason – for those thinking about pursuing this area as a subspeciality, this qualification can be very useful, both for your education and as evidence of your focus and ability. They may be attractive to those in anaesthesics, general practice, rheumatology, palliative medicine and many other specialities.

Obstetrics & Gynaecology

Advanced Gynaecological Endoscopy

* **Available levels:** MSc, PGDip, PGCert.
* **Available from:** University of Surrey.
* **Available through:** Part time.
* **Why do it?:** The course provides a theoretical grounding in gynaecological endoscopy as well as working alongside clinical training to develop operative

competence. It is relevant for both general O&G trainees and those considering a career in minimal-access surgery.

* **What it involves:** The course is composed of modules, each of which require several days' attendance. In addition operative experience is derived from the students' own department with an approved preceptor. Assessment is through written assignments and a logbook of cases with critical reflection. An OSCE is undertaken above PGCert level and the MSc requires an oral exam and a dissertation.
* **Is it worth it?:** Students report that the course not only develops their operative competence but also sorts out their clinical management of gynaecological conditions. It is dependent on obtaining enough clinical experience for the logbook however, which can be a problem with the current training scheme.

Ultrasound (O&G)

* **Available levels:** MSc, PGDip, PGCert.
* **Available from:** Bournemouth University, University of Cardiff.
* **Available through:** Full time, part time.
* **Why do it?:** Advanced scanning opportunities are difficult to come by in the current training environment. The courses offer a way to integrate scanning into your practice and, with the dissolution of the Diploma in Advanced Obstetric Ultrasound, offer one of the few ways to formalise your ultrasound training with a qualification.
* **What it involves:** The courses provide scientific grounding in the principles of ultrasound followed by focus on clinical O&G ultrasound. Both courses then require students to undertake ultrasound in their own department supervised by an approved trainer, producing a portfolio or logbook. A dissertation is required for the MSc.
* **Is it worth it?:** The courses offer an opportunity for advanced ultrasound training. This is particularly of interest for those planning a career in emergency gynaecology or fetal medicine. Remember though that the course depends on clinical experience being obtained in your own unit. This may be a problem if lack of available experience is why you are doing the course in the first place!

Paediatrics

Advanced Paediatrics, Child Health, Paediatrics and Child Health, Research Paediatrics, Paediatric Science, Community Paediatrics, Community Child Health, Tropical Paediatrics, Paediatric Infectious Disease, Child Public Health, International Child Health, Paediatric Diabetes, Paediatric Neurodisability

* **Available levels:** MSc, PGDip, PGCert.
* **Available from:** University College London; Universities of Leeds, Cardiff, Birmingham, Warwick, Nottingham, Oxford, Glasgow, Sheffield; Royal College of Paediatrics and Child Health; Liverpool School of Tropical Medicine.

* **Available through:** Full time or part time.
* **Why do it?:** All these courses provide a solid foundation in general paediatrics, but in addition may cover material not generally taught during routine paediatric training. They are generally available at various levels if you do not have the inclination or stamina to complete the dissertation to complete a master's, but there is flexibility to do this if your circumstances change. In the Yorkshire deanery in ST4–5, the Child Health master's/diploma is compulsory. The Diploma in Child Health (DCH) examination from the Royal College is a specific vocational qualification particularly aimed at general practice trainees.
* **What it involves:** Most of the institutions offering these courses require contact 1 day fortnightly for part-time students, although you can pick and choose modules for completion over up to a 5-year period. Some of the courses offer modules spread over the period of 1 week (which can be organised into a full-time course) to add up to 120 credits for a diploma. Those aiming for a master's degree will have to undertake a supervised research-based dissertation, which in most instances counts for 60 credits.
* **Is it worth it?:** Most of these courses encompass elements such as evidence-based medicine and statistics, leadership as well as specialist diagnoses, which may be appealing for those who are interested in these areas without necessarily doing a specific course. They can also provide evidence of advanced study in focussed areas of child health.

Psychiatry

Psychiatry, Clinical Psychiatry, Child and Adolescent Mental Health, Psychiatric Research, Clinical Neuropsychiatry

* **Available levels:** MSc, PGDip.
* **Available from:** Universities of Cardiff, Dundee, Leeds, Manchester, Sheffield, Liverpool, Northampton, King's College London, University College London.
* **Available through:** Full time or part time.
* **Why do it?:** These courses tend to be modular and can encompass areas such as psychopharmacology, neuropsychiatry and addiction, as well as core elements of evidence-based medicine, scientific methodology etc. Modules in psychotherapy, forensic psychiatry, old-age psychiatry and liaison psychiatry are optional.
* **What it involves:** Part-time students attend 1 day each week and can complete the courses over 2–3 years. Full-time students, have two timetabled days a week and the rest of the week in private study.
* **Is it worth it?:** The general psychiatry courses offer comprehensive coverage of sciences basic to psychiatry, critical appraisal, and theoretical and practical instruction in clinical psychiatry and its subspecialities. The research MSc is intended for psychiatry trainees who would wish to further their training in the research skills relevant to psychiatry and equip them with skills needed to begin doctoral level research.

Radiology

Radiology, Medical Diagnostics, Diagnostic Imaging,
Nuclear Medicine, MSc Endovascular Neurosurgery
(Interventional Neuroradiology)

* **Available levels:** MSc, PGDip.
* **Available from:** Universities of Cranfield, Oxford, Dundee, Canterbury, Salford, West of England, King's College Hospital, Royal College of Radiologists.
* **Available through:** Full time or part time over 2 years.
* **Why do it?:** The medical diagnostics course brings together biomedical and analytical science with production technology, business management, economics and ethics, thus allowing excellent expansion of non-medical skills. The diagnostic imaging course covers a vast range of areas within radiology from physics, to legislation regarding radiation and pharmacology.
* **What it involves:** Can be done full time or part time over 2–3 years. Teaching is based on lectures, but also small group teaching.
* **Is it worth it?:** Some of these courses are based on a 'core and options' structure, so you must anticipate a significant proportion of time spent in private study.

Summary

For those who wish to further their learning through a formal (taught) higher education course or degree, they can be an excellent way of expanding your knowledge in a field of your choice or interest. They can also provide formal evidence of the completion of learning in the relevant topic. However this pathway is not for all and the decision to undertake such courses is a complex one. As you have seen various factors (location, funding etc.) should be taken into account, and if you do pursue this avenue you will need to consider where this will take you in the future and what you hope to achieve. Do you wish this to be a one-off period of study? Or do you wish to use your master's, diploma or certificate as a springboard to a PhD or MD? If you are set on a career in academic medicine then it is more important to complete a research degree, and ideally a PhD, and this does not usually require a certificate or diploma as a prelude.

Whatever you wish to do in the future, a master's degree, diploma or certificate will enable you to gain new skills, further your knowledge and broaden your experiences, allowing for both personal and professional development.

The PhD

Susannah J Long
Andrew M Smith
M Justin S Zaman

◼ What is a PhD?

A PhD (sometimes DPhil) is a 'Doctor of Philosophy' and is the highest academic degree that can be gained. It is usually awarded after completion of a 3-year, full-time, period of original, high-quality research. It can take longer, and up to 6 years for part-time students. In the past the duration could lengthen but this is now strictly discouraged by pressure from funding bodies and universities. To be awarded a PhD you will need to complete a thesis or dissertation of your original academic research. This will be the longest essay you will ever write in your life and the contents must be worthy of publication in a peer-reviewed journal. You will need to defend your thesis in a viva voce (Latin for 'by live voice') examination to two examiners with expertise in the research area.

The core of a PhD is the application of deep and original thought on the fundamental principles of your chosen subject backed by high-quality novel evidence. This was indeed a main theme in ancient philosophy – ancient Greek philosophical tradition broke away from using mythology to explain the world, and instead offered an approach based on reason and evidence. PhDs offer 'research training' and having a PhD demonstrates that you have learnt and developed the necessary skills to be able to carry out novel research, analyse data and present your work to a high standard. Of course the expected outcome is that you will have also contributed a significant piece of new understanding to your chosen field. By their very nature PhDs are highly variable in terms of the types of research undertaken, the content and style of the thesis and expected outputs.

To undertake a PhD you will go through a rollercoaster of success and failure, often with rather more failure! This can be difficult for you, as a medical doctor, who is likely to have been successful in all academic pursuits thus far.

Three years is a long time and you must be motivated, passionate and have personal drive. Unlike clinical medicine where new patients, problems and solutions are dealt with daily, during a PhD you will often have prolonged periods where relatively little progress is made or anything concrete happens. You have to want to change something, or to delve into something you think is not adequately explained at the moment. Of course you can't do it yourself, but you can use your original ideas to find someone who can help you to explore your hypotheses. By completing a PhD as a clinician, you become an enquiring scientist usually with a passion for people and answering questions about disease, rather than a jobbing doctor who can remember long lists.

Alternative: MD

If you are less sure about 3 years of research (usually laboratory based), an MD is a shorter alternative and usually more clinically orientated. In the UK, MDs are postgraduate research degrees usually awarded after 2 years of research, which again has to be of a high standard, but of a smaller volume than for a PhD. Some projects are ideally suited for an MD, particularly if they are set up before you start, hopefully with research ethics approval already in place. Projects requiring more detailed exploration often of a more fundamental nature over a longer time frame are more suited to a PhD, particularly if the project is exploring a subject from scratch. Sometimes you may have the option of converting an MD to a PhD after the first year or so if it looks like another year of work might be useful (and if funding is available); it is best to check with your institution/supervisor before considering this though. For many an MD will be a good alternative. However if your aspirations are to be a full-time clinical academic, aiming for a professorial position ultimately, or at least a senior research fellowship, then a PhD in a subject linked to basic science research is likely to be more useful.

Why should doctors do a PhD/MD?

People tend to undertake postgraduate studies for one of three reasons:

1 **An academic/medical interest** – Taking a PhD is the first step on a career path in academic medicine. A PhD will give you the full flavour of what medical research entails and how it progresses, and therefore whether a future in academic medicine is indeed for you. To undertake a PhD you will undoubtedly be interested in your subject and will be striving to discover new ideas and concepts. For some students this may be the opportunity they have longed for: to research an area that has either been of personal interest or one that lies undiscovered. You may think for instance that a certain drug does not work as well in a particular group of patients, and that some form of pharmaco-genetic study may improve the targeting of whom might benefit. Or you might just know you are keen to explore the underlying causes of a disease, and get excited by the prospects your supervisor suggests. It is

certainly possible to make new breakthroughs and be the first to find something, though time restrictions will limit this. However, your PhD can be a stepping stone for further discovery. Certainly some people have been able to patent their discoveries (along with their funding bodies and university) and write *Nature* or *Science* papers as a result of their research. This may lead to financial reward, but you should not start a PhD in the hope of this as the chances are remote. Finally, remember undertaking a PhD is still a form of training – research training.

2 **Employment prospects** – People may choose to do a PhD/MD to enhance their career prospects. Attaining a PhD shows future employers that you possess a number of valuable skills such as self-motivation, dedication and enthusiasm, as well as academic and intellectual abilities. You may find that some highly competitive posts at academic institutions or teaching hospitals require postgraduate qualifications as an essential criterion. Geography plays a large role, with large hospitals in major cities often only taking on consultants with PhDs/MDs. In the past, some registrar training posts could only be attained with a higher degree, but this is now much less common. Remember, if this is your primary driver, you may quickly get frustrated and bored if you've not chosen your subject carefully.

3 **Personal challenge** – Some doctors take on this form of study to prove to themselves that they are capable of completing it. To complete a PhD successfully you will need to be highly motivated and exceptionally enthusiastic.

Personal perspective by Dr Zaman

I originally aspired to be an interventional cardiologist, but when I moved to a hospital in a deprived city area I saw the influence of social inequality on disease. Unhealthy lifestyles increased the likelihood of ischaemic heart disease but also deprivation reduced the likelihood of patients staying healthy after treatment. I realised that health promotion was poorly delivered in deprived areas and that societal changes could influence disease and treatment. So my reason for wanting to undertake research, and ultimately a PhD, was a personal passion to change what I saw as an inequity in medicine. I could also see a way to finding an answer to my question – and that is important, as you will want to have a result at the end of the PhD! Having this personal desire to answer a question you see in front of you will also make the 3-plus years less painful. A PhD is not easy but if you can take your mind to your 'ground zero' inspiration moment, it will pull you through.

Is a PhD for me?

If you have a genuine interest and curiosity in a particular subject, you are a determined individual and you feel able to dedicate the necessary 3 or 4 years of your life, you should definitely consider doing a PhD in our view. Certainly this is true if you want ultimately to consider a career in academic medicine. If you are the type of person who always asks why and is never fully satisfied until you have all the facts about a particular question, then you are ideally suited to a PhD studentship. It is crucial to have an inquisitive and open mind in order to produce the original research required to attain a PhD. Unlike all other examinations you have ever undertaken the PhD is about discovering and understanding complex problems in which the answers are not available in textbooks. This can be an exhilarating and frustrating experience for most and a major stumbling block for some. The time taken to achieve a PhD is considerable but restricted (the 3 years will go very fast), therefore make sure you can commit for the full duration of the course. Research can be a lonely and frustrating business. The majority of time you will be working independently and under your own initiative, which can be difficult to get used to. Previous experience within a laboratory will prove invaluable and help you decide if you are capable of lasting the course.

For people pursuing academic careers in scientific disciplines outside of medicine (such as pure biochemistry or pharmacology), doing a PhD often follows on quickly and naturally from earlier degrees, and is seen as the first real step in becoming an independent researcher. In medicine, the usual pattern is to concentrate on clinical training first, then venture into the world of academia at a later stage. This means that by the time most doctors do a PhD they already have considerable life experience, maturity and a sense of responsibility: it could be argued that all of these attributes make for better research. Conversely, PhD students are older, more encumbered socially, and have more rigid brains further from a time spent learning basic science at university! The downside of this, though, is the steeper learning curve in acquiring research skills compared to scientists in other fields. However this is not insurmountable – there are plenty of sources of support and learning resources for doctors who are new to research. Similarly, developing a sound set of research skills can bring benefits to your clinical practice, enabling you to better appraise published work and clinical evidence and reflect on your clinical practice.

Overview of PhD process

The process will vary according to the type of project you undertake. Many of the early activities will overlap the process of gaining a personal research fellowship:

* An extensive literature search of your subject.
* Choose your supervisor(s).
* Choose your location (university/hospital/department/laboratory/research group). Your supervisor and the research group are fundamentally important to a successful PhD. You need a supervisor with time and a track

record of success, and a research group also with a track record of successful research, grants, publications and previous successful PhD students.

* Identify any collaborators you may need, and technical input (e.g. statistician).
* Have a broad idea of the body of your thesis – i.e. the main research chapters and hence the potential papers – these will be your main research projects, and you will need about 3–4 big 'experiments' to provide enough weight for a PhD. You will have discussed this in your planning of the PhD with your supervisor.
* Research training in techniques required to undertake the project.
* You may need to achieve other educational targets during the 3 years depending on local conditions, e.g. your university may require you to undertake training in research management and ethics by attending internal courses.
* Ethical approval may be required for your work, which you may need to lead.
* Once started, there will be an 'upgrade' process at 1 year as all PhD candidates start as MPhil students – you will need to nominate an examiner for this, usually external to your university.
* The first year will be when you do at least one of the main experiments of the PhD to prepare for your upgrade process, whilst also laying the foundations of the other experiments.
* The second year is when you will do the main bulk of the experiments, and also put together abstracts for presentation at scientific conferences based on your results.
* The final year will involve completing your research and the writing of the main papers – and hence the main chapters of your thesis – and putting it all together into one dissertation.
* The final examination is the viva examination of your thesis, and you will need to have nominated two examiners in good time prior to the viva, at least one external to the university.

Inevitably time pressure catches up with everyone as the following occur frequently: (1) research almost never goes exactly to plan and experiments never go right first time; (2) other research groups publish the same work you are doing; (3) funding does not materialise; (4) reagents and data sets are not available as expected; (5) you get sidetracked or (6) your time is too stretched by interesting clinical demands.

Choosing your project

The field

PhD studies can incorporate almost anything, so you must spend time thinking about research areas that interest you. Like everything in life, scientific research is governed by fashion and there are always topics that are in and out of favour. This means that funding and studentships are usually more readily available in certain fields and equally, it can seem almost impossible to obtain funding in less fashionable topics. Things are not static and fashions will change during your PhD. Therefore, take this ever-changing background into consideration when choosing potential study areas. You can get an idea of the current hot research areas by looking at the lists of funded grants available on all major grant bodies' websites. A key consideration though is the track record of the research group and supervisor you would be working with in obtaining grants, and developing a project closely with your supervisor.

Clinical or laboratory

Once you have identified a broad research interest, then consider whether you want to do 'clinical' or 'laboratory'-based research, or a combination of both. In reality combining both and completing high-quality original research in the time available is extremely difficult. Obviously some of the skills that you will be required to learn in these different types of research will be very different, particularly in terms of methodology. In either case, it is helpful and important always to keep in mind the clinical relevance of your work – this will after all be the underlying reason why you are doing the research in the first place. Some consider clinical research as 'dirty' because there are so many variables and confounders that simply cannot be accounted for. Furthermore, you will need to find patients to enrol and convince them that it is worth participating in your work. This is harder than it sounds! Some consider a laboratory-based PhD as more 'pure' as it generally involves more basic science, answers more fundamental questions with potentially wider remit, and you can (in theory) control all the variables within an experiment. However it can feel quite removed from clinical work and may pigeonhole you as a 'scientist' rather than a clinician.

Ultimately the choice of clinical or laboratory research will depend on you and how you view things. Both have great potential and both will require you to exploit fully all the options available. Translational research is an increasingly popular type of research in which emphasis is the application of 'bench' research to the 'bedside'. How this is done will depend entirely on your field and project. Clearly if you can't face 3 years in a laboratory dealing with cells, molecules, mice or tissue sections then a laboratory-based PhD is not for you. If you can get a taster of such work then this may help you make up your mind (see Chapters 2 and 3 on academic clinical fellowships). Ultimately however if you think you may want to pursue an academic career you will need to have undertaken a PhD achieving high-quality results, and those choosing to answer more fundamental questions in general are more likely to achieve the most academic success in the long run.

Key points

Choosing your PhD can involve many factors. Consider the following:
- **Interest:** You must be interested (ideally passionate and excited) about your project. This will sustain you through it. A lack of interest will only intensify over 3 years!

- **Your suitability:** Does the project feature things that you're good at or can learn? Make sure it matches your skill base, or will train you in a set of skills you are interested in obtaining (e.g. echocardiography in a cardiology PhD). Consider whether you can work with animals or abroad if that is required as part of the project
- **Suitability of your supervisor:** Is the project within the supervisor's research field? Have they got publications in this field, or is it a new venture? If it's new, do they have realistic aims? Have they supervised PhD students before? Have they won grant funding recently?
- **Feasibility of the research:** Can you actually do your project in that environment? For example for basic science work does the lab have the right reagents and equipment? Is there space to assess patients for clinical work? Is the question simply too big to be answered in the 3 years? Is the timeframe for the project realistic and does it allow enough time for mistakes and errors? All of these questions will need to be answered to funding bodies as well
- **Who else will be working on the project?** It's likely you'll be working as part of a larger research group. Find out how closely you'll be working with others. You'll need to establish boundaries and ensure your work is independent

Applying for your PhD

Once you have chosen your broad field of interest, you will need to undertake a literature search to ensure the answer is not already out there! Doing this will also highlight the big names in the field. Make a shortlist and consider their background – the speciality they are in does not need to be the same as yours, but you may prefer that. Check the institution they work in – is there a broader interest within the department or university for the subject, and hence a research infrastructure and potential for collaboration and wider support? Does the institution have a track record of high-quality research output? You may prefer to stay local to where you are currently based, but in general you should go to where you think the best PhD can be undertaken (and consider going overseas). Your colleagues may also recommend potential research groups, or you may be aware of an institution or research group where you would like to work. Don't forget basic science laboratories of which your clinical colleagues may be less aware – ask around widely.

You now have two main options – approaching supervisors directly or responding to an advertised post:

1 **Applying independently to a specific department** – Contact a potential supervisor directory and ask about research opportunities. Once approached, departments are usually glad to meet and discuss new ideas and possible future collaborations. Remember, it is in their interests to have new PhD students as it will bring new income and funding to their department,

hopefully publications and potentially a new direction to take their research interests. These meetings will therefore be a two-way process; you can see if their interests match yours, and they can assess you as a potential PhD candidate. If the discussion is fruitful and it seems possible that you might join the group to undertake a PhD, you and your potential supervisor will need to work out a suitable timeframe and apply for funding. You may have to complete a piece of work to demonstrate your commitment, or work in that 'lab' to gain experience with that particular group. Gaining any laboratory experience will be invaluable in any grant applications or interviews. Ultimately your supervisor will suggest applying for a research training fellowship, e.g. from the Wellcome Trust or MRC, or may (unusually) have access to funding independently.

2 **Responding to an advert** – Sometimes you can apply for projects that are already set up by an experienced academic (who will usually be your supervisor), either with partial or complete funding. These research posts are then advertised for example in the British Medical Journal or on the websites of specialist medical societies. If funding is not available for the whole PhD when it starts you may have to apply for further funding after 1–2 years. This is less than ideal since there is no guarantee of funding to project (PhD) completion. Ideally, the project you end up doing should be something that you can feel passionate about and something that fits in with your long-term career interests. You should ensure that the simplicity of applying for a ready-made post doesn't mean you end up undertaking a project that is of no interest to you.

Impressing your potential supervisor

Your potential supervisor will be a key person in your life for the next 3–5 years and may influence your future over the next decade! Impressing them early will help you. Your past academic record will clearly be a major factor. Ensure your CV is ready for a PhD application. Get involved in any publications (e.g. as a 'middle' author), write a case report or editorial review, and revise the project you may have done as an intercalated BSc student and how that gave you a first taste of research. Perhaps go on a 'research methods' course, although this is less helpful. If you have nothing on your CV to show academic ability you will not get funding nor any chance of undertaking a PhD!

Beyond that it comes down to your drive and enthusiasm. A potential supervisor wants to see a spark in a potential student, a true passion for the subject. Tell them how you have investigated the research field concerning the subject so far. Elaborate on how you think that the project might make true scientific progress and how it might impact on future clinical practice (where relevant). A potential supervisor will almost certainly not want you to have come up with specific research questions and plans, but clearly you will impress if you have thought about these. This may simply entail a broad hypothesis (e.g. why do some ethnic groups have a higher incidence of a particular disease, and is this due to a difference in genes or a difference in environment) and some detail on how you might study it (e.g. use the supervisor's cohort study of patients with that disease). Perhaps discuss what you might come up with by the end, and how you foresee it changing practice.

Key points

- Visit at least a couple of potential supervisors, even if you are convinced by your top choice
- Ask about the success rate of previous PhDs
- Emphasise your ideas and integrate these into your planned project whilst intertwining the current work being undertaken by your supervisor and perhaps ideas of collaborating with other departments in that university
- Project ideas should evolve through discussion. Once you have both accepted each other (and it is a two-way process) then detailed planning will begin on the research project

---

Tell them how you found them and why they and the work they are doing is pivotal to what you want to achieve. You may also talk about the importance of the institution. Be honest if you have already seen other potential supervisors and what you thought their advantages and disadvantages.

Once you think you have found the right supervisor, your joint ideas and hypotheses will grow into something that is scientifically achievable, feasible for you to conduct, and realistic to conclude and you can now begin applying for funding.

Pitfall

Don't necessarily chase the biggest name in the field. An international leader may not be able to give you the time you will need. You should visit if they offer you a chance, but be wary. The best supervisor may be someone 'up and coming' whose own head of department is a true leader in the field. Regular time with a supervisor is crucial.

Pitfall

- Tell supervisors who else you have met! Be honest because the world is small and they may be good friends.
- If you're declining a potential supervisor, do so in a polite, courteous and professional manner. People have egos and these bruise easily if rejected in a bad way. Think hard and explain why you are going elsewhere. Don't have silent doubts and pull this out later; this will annoy and frustrate supervisors who have put time into you.

Role of supervisors

PhD students can have one or two supervisors, two becoming increasingly common. They are there to guide and support you through the process of doing the PhD and ensure that your work meets the required standards. Your university will have its own rules about who these people might be. Usually your principle supervisor will be based in your research department, and will have previous experience in PhD supervision. A second supervisor may be more of an academic mentor, or to maintain clinical links, and may be from outside the department or speciality. It can be very helpful to have supervisors from different backgrounds, for example one pure academic and one a clinical academic, so you will have the best of both worlds in terms of academic learning and support and somebody to make sure that what you are doing remains clinically relevant and useful to your future. This may not always be appropriate.

Rarely you may find that to 'cover all the bases' your project even requires three supervisors – the third person may for example be an expert in an entirely different discipline, such as business or technology. The main thing is that you find a good balance of supervisors if you have more than one, and ideally a combination of personalities and viewpoints. However, make sure that you can regularly meet the other supervisors and they are not just names on the paperwork! Most supervisors have many areas of interest and they may be supervising several other PhD students. Some supervisors are simply more productive than others but consider carefully if they will have time for you.

Key point

- Think about having a primary and a secondary supervisor, in *differing* but complementary fields. You will get more supervision, differing perspectives and a multidisciplinary approach, which is so important in contemporary research.

At the beginning of the project the principle supervisor's role will be critical, but as the programme develops the student will take the initiative, reducing the need for direct supervision. Towards the end more supervision will be required for 'writing up'. The process of supervision will develop at different speeds depending on the ability of both the supervisor and student.

The desirable attributes of a good supervisor, whatever their field of expertise, are: (1) a genuine interest in you and your work, (2) approachability, (3) the time that you will need with them, (4) an ability to provide you with constructive criticism, and obviously (5) a strong academic background in the field of the research and ideally wide collaborations. It is important that they are someone with whom you can get on and feel able to talk openly. Sometimes you may feel that your ideas sound silly and you need someone who will keep an open mind and will help and encourage you to develop. They also need to be experienced at supervising, and be aware of the relevant procedures and rules within your institution. You should also check that their previous PhD students have completed their projects in the allotted time.

When meeting potential supervisors, consider how similar your personalities are. Also, meet other members of the research team – if they are happy, then it is likely there is a happy research environment. Try to meet them alone to understand their first-hand views and seek an unbiased opinion. Beware though, some of those you speak to, may be entering the 'disillusioned' phase of their PhD (often in the second year!) so be cautious of overly pessimistic views.

Funding

If you are lucky, you will find a suitable project that already has funding. This is rare. In most instances you will need to apply for funding, usually in the form of a research training fellowship to pay your salary for 3 years and possibly some research or ancillary costs. This can be a long process; you will need to start preparing for this a year in advance and you will need a lot of help from your supervisors. Your funding proposal should show the importance and justification of what it is that you wish to achieve, be based on solid scientific work, and the proposed methodology will need to be robust. Judgement will be based on you, your project and the host department/research group/supervisor.

There are several sources of funding and your supervisor will be the best person to advise you on this. Some large organisations such as the Medical Research Council or the National Institute for Health Research have specific funding streams for clinical or research training fellowships, designed for doctors in training to undertake a PhD. Other organisations that may be able to offer help include relevant charitable organisations or specialist medical societies. It may be that you only obtain funding for the first year or so at the first go: you will then need to apply for further money based on your initial findings and scope for further work. Funding, grant proposals and the interviews required for this are covered in detail in Chapters 6 and 9.

Doing your PhD

First steps

Once you have funding you will need to take time out of your clinical training programme, by applying for time 'out-of-programme for research' (OOPR) through your deanery. This is the usual process if you are already a SpR or an ST3 or above, or in a run-through training programme such as paediatrics or psychiatry. Discuss this early with your training programme director, and before you even apply for funding. If you've chosen to do your research earlier, such as after FY2 or CT2 in core medicine for example, then seek deanery advice but you may not need formal approval since you are not taking time out from within a training programme.

Your deanery website will tell you how to do this, but in general you will need the approval of your training programme director and educational supervisor, and dean or head of speciality school. If you want any of the research time to count towards your CCT (usually up to 1 year is allowed), you must apply to the relevant Royal College (for example the JRCPTB of the Royal College of Physicians), and you will also need GMC approval of your post. Once you have all of this, and you have been appointed to your research post, there are several procedures that need to be followed, the details of which will vary depending on the university.

A common process involves registering with the university for an MPhil initially in most cases, for which you will need to submit a research plan that has been assessed by two individuals (not your supervisors). After about 12–18 months you undergo an 'MPhil to PhD transfer' process ('upgrade'), which checks that your doctoral project is on track, viable and that you are capable of completing it successfully. This varies between universities but generally entails submitting a written report of the work you have completed to date, or a written project that is agreed locally. You may then have two assessors conduct your viva (one internal to the university and one external) or have to make a formal presentation. This is an invaluable opportunity to gain feedback on the work you have done so far and your plans for the rest of the PhD from outside your immediate research group. This can be scary and but if done correctly can help the rest of the PhD fly. Your examiners will provide a detailed review of your submission and you can use this to support your next 2 years. If successful you will be transferred to full PhD registration.

Your university may also allocate a PhD mentor completely separate from your project who can help independently of your research group. The final formal procedure at the end of the PhD is thesis submission after selection of examiners.

Personal perspective of upgrading by Dr Zaman

"I chose a highly critical and eminent external name in my field as my external examiner for my upgrade. My supervisor felt it would be better to meet him at this stage rather than the final viva! He was unbelievably thorough, and provided an incredibly critical and useful review after which my PhD flew – though clearly the viva was not fun! I had a detailed account of one experiment within a 10 000-word dissertation as well as the skeletal outlines of my other three main experiments to demonstrate that the PhD would eventually come together as one coherent argument. I also gave a presentation to the department".

Early days

Start the first week by sitting with your supervisor and writing a 6-month plan of initial objectives, as well as a rough PhD contents page outlining the chapters you might eventually write. It may seem a long way off, but it helps to start thinking of this as a coordinated and logical project. Borrow a PhD dissertation from someone to get an idea of the format. Make sure you plan things you need to do by certain times – the first few weeks may seem like a holiday compared to being on the wards, but that will not last! Early on in your PhD, plan how you will spend your 3 years, and keep updating this plan, ensuring you are keeping to time.

In particular, get on with the literature search. Be careful to document all your searches as you may need to reproduce them both later and in your dissertation. File important background literature in a logical way on your hard drive so you can retrieve them easily, e.g. label with the author name first, then title, then year. Back everything up on a different computer. Collect references in full, not just the abstract. As a PhD student and budding career academic you should learn to read the methods section of other investigators' papers first.

Being organised is a key skill needed when undertaking a PhD. Use a diary as the last thing you want to do is miss a meeting with a research collaborator! Take the chance to go on the free staff development courses that exist locally, which will enhance you, your research abilities and your CV. Most universities will stipulate this as part of the process and have set courses you need to complete.

Arrange regular meetings with your supervisor – monthly initially as a minimum – and set an agenda each time with resulting action points. Minute them and file them since this will act like a research diary. A good supervisor will provide regular, constructive criticism on your written work, guidance, suggestions and ideas for research avenues, help with the literature and direction. In return, you should show initiative and be proactive as you must eventually become independent, and be honest as to how things are going and whether you are struggling with any aspect. Produce high-quality written work when writing abstracts or papers that does not look like a messy first draft and meet deadlines.

Years 2 and 3

Once past the 'upgrade', you must aim to get your main experiments done during your second year. Hopefully by then you will be familiar with most of the research methods you will need. Stick to the major three to four you had planned and don't be tempted to do 'small-fry' side-projects. You must focus on a few core research questions and not dilute the PhD with lots of small experiments. Less is more! Write abstracts as you go along and submit them to national and international conferences. When writing abstracts, sketch out the paper first. Aim never to submit an abstract without it becoming a paper eventually. This will make for a more coherent and successful abstract and makes for better science. The papers will also effectively be your main research chapters for the thesis and will make the writing up in your final year much easier. All of your main experiments should ideally result in abstract presentation at a conference. At conferences use the abstract (be it in the form of a poster or presentation) to network and search for future potential collaborators – your PhD will eventually end, and you will need to find more work! Make a business card for yourself.

The final year should entail the submission and hopefully publication of at least two of your experiments as full papers, and the writing of the thesis. Ensure you have also looked into the submission details, in particular the deadlines! Read every word on the university website carefully on administration of the PhD – your supervisor may not know all the details, and it is your job to check this. It is your thesis after all. Start to think about who you will want to examine you with your supervisor, and give your supervisor the names and contact details for them to contact in plenty of time. It is crucial that you finish your thesis completely before returning to full-time clinical work. There is a temptation to believe you can write up the thesis in evenings and weekends but in reality this is extremely difficult. Furthermore many universities will now impose penalties on students who do not complete fully within 3 years as they are under pressure from governmental funding agencies to show students completing higher degrees.

What skills can I expect to gain?

You have to be disciplined, self-sufficient and have enough initiative to find answers yourself to problems you might encounter. You may need to learn many practical or technical skills from the scientists and academics you are working with. You will probably need to gain expertise in a range of qualitative and quantitative methodologies and your university will most likely provide a range of free courses that you can attend. Some of these courses will in fact be mandatory, such as health and safety, radiation safety, and animal handling, but even a course in writing skills, time management, ethics, basic statistics and more. Depending on where you work, such courses will be open to PhD students in all subjects, giving you another opportunity to learn from students in various disciplines and with different backgrounds.

Key points

- Remember a PhD is training in how to do research: ensure you learn basic research methodology
- Take time to understand and learn laboratory techniques or clinical skills – you take this beyond your PhD
- Learn how to write effectively in a scientific manner

As well as technical research skills, completing a PhD will also allow you to develop more generic skills that will be useful throughout your career, whether or not you stay in academia. For example research involves a great deal of teamworking and collaboration and your writing, presentation and IT skills will undoubtedly also be enhanced.

Practicalities

You should make full use of the many other facilities and resources that will be available to you such as excellent library services with on-line access to thousands of journal articles, statistical advisory services, seminars and lectures from visiting scholars to different departments, and training in teaching, to name but a few.

There are of course some practical disadvantages to doing a PhD, such as the reduction in income. This can be quite significant since you will normally be paid an unbanded salary at your current NHS level. You may be able to supplement this income by doing locum work, or being part of an on-call rota at weekends or evenings, but it is crucial you don't let this impinge on your research time, which of course is why you are doing your PhD. You should also be aware that as a clinician undertaking research you are undoubtedly earning much more than any pure scientists in the laboratory or group doing similar (or even higher level) work.

Settling into the lifestyle of a PhD student is also a shock to clinicians. If you have come from a busy clinical job, starting a full-time PhD can be very strange, with more flexible working hours, fewer structured days, and of course without your bleep! You will be working in a completely new environment, perhaps being based in an office or laboratory for the first time in your life. However the pressures and responsibilities of clinical work are soon replaced by the demands of the research, which always takes much much longer than you might think.

The rollercoaster

There is massive variation between PhD programmes. You may come racing out of the starting blocks and begin collecting data straightaway. In contrast, some projects have huge teething problems and seem to be going nowhere for months. Remember that even if a colleague seems to be getting on better then you, every project will have ups and downs.

Mistakes are common in the first few months and may lead to frustration. Recognise that these are normal and you will improve very quickly. You can speed your learning curve by working closely with an experienced researcher and ask as many questions as possible. It is safer to ask for help than to try and blunder along regardless. Don't forget that laboratories can be dangerous so work safely!

It is essential you work to realistic timetables and deadlines. Your supervisors will of course give you regular feedback on your work. They will probably also be required to complete formal progress reports on a 6-monthly basis and there will also be an opportunity for you confidentially to raise any concerns about your supervisors. You will also have annual assessments by your deanery (at an academic ARCP), at which you will be expected to submit progress reports from your supervisor.

You and your supervisor

What you can expect from them

* Regular supervision meetings to discuss your work and progress.
* Seek new approaches or directions for your work.
* Advice on designing studies.
* Help you write articles for publication.
* Help with your thesis.

The frequency and length of your supervision meetings will vary during the course of your PhD. You will need most support at the beginning and towards the end of your research. You should be able to feel free to contact your supervisors for advice in between meetings. It is also advisable to arrange joint meetings with all your supervisors occasionally (if you have more than one) so consensus can be reached if there are differing views about your work and joint plans can be made.

What they will expect from you

* Hard work! Research does not fit into a 9–5 day.
* Showing initiative.
* Taking on board feedback.
* Behaving in a professional, honest and responsible way – you will after all be representing them and their department in any contact you have with the outside world, whether through written publications or conference presentations.
* Being involved in other output from the research group.
* Your help with other work within the department, for example helping to apply for funding, or providing advice and support for other researchers within your department as you become more experienced.

Other activities during the PhD

In order to ensure your focus is not too narrow and to maintain your professional development, it's a good idea to try to get involved with some other activities during your PhD. However you must stay focused on your own thesis, and a PhD is a more than full-time occupation in its own right.

> **Key point**
> * Make the most of opportunities presented to you but don't make promises you can't keep or let sideline projects distract you too much from your PhD work.

* **Research/academic activities** – Some of these will be directly related to your PhD, such as presenting at departmental meetings or national/international conferences. Attend seminars and lectures in your department and find out

if any similar departments in other universities have open-access events. Discuss your work with visiting academics, who may well come from abroad. Over the 3 years you will build a network of contacts that may well be useful in the short or long term. You may be invited to visit other departments, participate in other research projects or to contribute to joint publications. You can become a peer reviewer for a journal, reading papers submitted and considering them for publication.

* **Non-academic activities** – You might be able to get involved in regular undergraduate medical teaching (and examining) locally, or regular clinical teaching for postgraduate exams such as the MRCP. You might be asked to teach on BSc or MSc courses in relation to your PhD project or the techniques you use. Your university will probably offer formal teaching courses, perhaps leading to postgraduate qualifications. This is a great opportunity as your timetable will be more flexible than during clinical jobs.

* **Clinical role** – It is important to maintain your links with clinical practice during the 3-year period but not to get too distracted by what can often seem the 'safe haven' of clinical work. You may have timetabled clinical sessions during your PhD and you will almost certainly have an honorary clinical contract if your research is clinically based. Formal clinical sessions such as an outpatient clinic should not occupy more than half a day per week if at all possible, and ideally none in your first year. If you want to work extra clinical shifts (to 'keep your hand in' and supplement your income), find out if you can join your hospital's bank of locum staff (the ideal option) or join a locum agency. This must not compromise your research time though. Keep going to your regional training days if not too frequent, and any clinical conferences or meetings as these will help you to keep in touch with the clinical world and with your peers.

Key points

Try to keep in touch with your clinical world. If you do not have timetabled clinical sessions, join your hospitals locum bank. Try not to do more than one clinical session per week (e.g. one outpatient clinic) and locum work ideally only at weekends. The PhD is a full-time occupation. Keep going to regional training days and clinical meetings and conferences.

Your thesis

The structure of your thesis will of course depend on the type of work you have done. In general, though, the main principle is that the thesis should flow, almost like a story of your research, starting with an introduction to your topic, leading to a justification of your hypotheses, how you went about testing them, the findings, and their significance. People have different views about whether it is best to write your thesis 'as you go along', or at the end of your research.

You will of course be writing during the course of your research anyway for your MPhil-PhD transfer report and for any publications or grant applications. It takes time for the flow of your research to develop into well-formulated ideas and conclusions, so many people spend the last 12 months of their PhD 'writing up'. It can be helpful to get feedback from other people (such as interested colleagues), in addition to your supervisors, during this time (if you can get agreement from them to do this). It is helpful to plan the reading with your supervisors and other reviewers: you may wish to send different chapters to different individuals at different times to spread the workload. Reading thesis chapters intelligently and critically is not easy!

Thesis writing is probably the hardest part of a PhD for the majority of students and it is commonly feared by PhD students. The style of writing and the need to inject enthusiasm into the thesis after 3 years of research work can be difficult. Furthermore, it will take time and dedication and will be the largest body of work you'll produce. However, if you look to enjoy the writing process and consider it a chance to prove all your efforts over the 3 years, it will be easier. To ensure you finish within a good time, set yourself a submission date and be strict with yourself.

Pitfall

Watch out for plagiarism. This can be in the form of copied text, images and using results from other laboratory members. Inclusion of all these are acceptable in moderation as long as the credit is given to the original source and no attempt is made to take personal credit.

An example contents page from a thesis is shown in Figure 8.1.

In this example, chapters 5 to 8 were the four main 'experiments'. Chapter 9 aimed to bring together the previous four chapters into one logical argument prior to the Discussion. The answers in this 'summation' chapter were in response to the initial questions at the beginning of the introduction, whilst the rest of the introduction sought to present the rationale behind the ensuing main experiments.

Write your main experimental chapters in a consistent fashion, and model them as scientific papers. However, be more critical than is usual in a paper on your methodology. Try to predict what criticisms your examiners will eventually come up with! Make sure your tables and figures are also consistent in their design, and are labelled logically, i.e. numbered '5.3' if part of chapter 5, and the titles have a similar style throughout. Are the figures clear and can you understand the message from them without reading the accompanying text? Do not write overlong and complex sentences.

The thesis must logically flow. Right from page 1, it must be clear how the original question leads to a logical and relevant literature review, and that in turn to a logical experiment that answers that question and that question alone.

Figure 8.1 Sample thesis contents page

If your experiment did come up with an unexpected but interesting relevant finding, then you must lay the rationale down for that in the introduction! Presenting it naively within the chapter of the experiment is not the way to do it! Any ideas that you cannot answer could be presented under 'Future directions' in your Discussion chapter rather than in the Introduction. Your experiments may have uncovered many other interesting avenues. These can then be your Aims and Objectives and then be explained in your discussion.

Finally, don't worry about the word count. You will have plenty to say.

The viva

When you are near completion you will need to discuss potential examiners with your supervisors. The formal requirement will usually be for two examiners, one from within your university but outside your department and one completely external. It is important that your examiners are familiar with the research area and have sufficient time to read the thesis. Check with your university regulations as rules may differ. You will need to complete submission forms to your university registry well in advance.

Most students fear the actual viva voce more than anything else, but really should not! You will never experience a more gruelling academic examination in your life but remember that you will know more than your examiners on the specific topic of your PhD! The viva voce examination is essentially a detailed discussion of your work in which you will be required to justify and explain your methods, results and conclusions. The examiners must check carefully that your conclusions are valid by scrutinising your methodology and that your work is original and important. Consider it as a discussion with two bright people above you in the research food chain that are genuinely interested in your work and want it to be correct.

The examiners will start with an open question asking you to summarise what you did over 3 years and you must have practiced this answer. After this initial question (where you should hopefully shine), the examiners will start to cross-examine you. In preparing do not try to predict other questions, but instead go through the thesis a number of times and think back to how the research evolved. Recall your supervisor's own lines of criticism. Stay calm, confident and professional. Take time to answer. Do not become visibly angry or arrogant, but instead compliment the examiners (occasionally!) on picking up the arcane or subtle points, and be rigorous and methodological in your line of answering.

If an examiner has a concern about an important omitted fact or argument then accept that it would have been good to have included it. However, have a ready defence as to why it was not possible, and how your argument still stands in the most part. Try suggesting that it is an area for future research.

As well as knowing all of the work within your thesis and all the referenced papers, it is also a good idea to read up on the examiners' own publications. It is amazing how often examiners resort to asking questions closely associated with their own work and ignorance on the part of the PhD student will only aggravate and prolong the viva. In some cases the viva can be a substantial time after the submission of the thesis and the candidate may have started another job. In these circumstances it is important to keep up to date with the published literature and your research group's research. On the whole a viva examination will last between 2 and 4 hours. Your supervisor may wish to sit in during the examination but this is not necessary and may distract you.

The viva ends with the examiners making one of four decisions:

1 **Accepted without any corrections** – This would be the ideal outcome – the thesis is accepted as presented and you are awarded the PhD. Unfortunately this is not common, as the examiners will feel they have something to contribute! If you get this outcome, it's time to open the champagne and have a party!
2 **Accepted with minor corrections or revision** – This is the most common decision. In general the revisions will be clarification of concepts or methodology. Changes in the field may necessitate addition of sections. Sometimes clarification of figures or tables or their legends, or statistical

analysis is required. Once these are made one of the examiners will assess the revisions and provide written confirmation that they have been satisfactorily completed.

3 **Extensive revision required before re-evaluation** – This may occur if you have not sought help with your thesis and it has become a muddled document. You will need to make extensive changes, and whilst disheartening, it may be worth taking a fresh stab at it. Seek help from your supervisor immediately. If you had a good rapport with your supervisor, meeting regularly including mid-point assessments, this outcome should not occur. Once resubmitted, you have a second viva with the same examiners. If your fail this, then you will need to withdraw from the PhD programme.

4 **Unacceptable thesis** – This is the worst possible outcome and is a bad end of a long journey. This means that the examiners don't feel you can make changes necessary to save the thesis, or that you demonstrated poor knowledge of your work, it lacked originality or was insufficient in quality. Unfortunately you will have to withdraw from the PhD programme and cannot resubmit.

Life after your PhD

Planning for this needs to start during your PhD! What happens next really depends on you, whether you have enjoyed the research, the stage of your career and your long-term career plans. Many people decide to combine a clinical and academic career after their PhD. Exactly how this is achieved will vary, but you will undoubtedly need to apply for further grants, lectureships or fellowships, and continue to develop your research ideas and skills. If you have enjoyed the research and there is a chance to write a post-doctoral grant proposal with your supervisor, seize it. Equally, seek and assess how you might be able to undertake post-doctoral work in another department as movement outwards will broaden your experience prior to a senior lectureship post.

The key academic pathways following a PhD for medically trained researchers are CLs and intermediate fellowships. Ensure that post-doctoral work is planned early such that you will have the time to accrue the CV required to apply for these awards. Make sure you finish the papers from the PhD! This is key to showing that you are a 'finisher'. Ask your supervisor to be honest in your likelihood of winning such posts, especially intermediate fellowships, or better still senior colleagues from other departments who sit on grant-giving committees.

Show off and highlight your work. You are now a bona fide academic! Write letters to journals addressing points in articles on similar work to yours, reviews or editorials, and cite your own work within. This may lead to future collaborations. You are aiming possibly for a Chair and need to get a lecturer and then senior lecturer position first (and finish clinical training). So there is still a long way to go. If you wish, are academically successful and are lucky, you may be able to train clinically 50% and continue research the rest of the time in posts such as CLs. Unlike clinical medicine, where a consultancy or GP principal seems to represent a target to many, research is more about the journey, not the destination. The more you seek answers, the more questions you will unravel as an academic. You will – if your original passion was strong and genuine – never lose the desire to experiment.

You may choose to return to purely clinical work and use the PhD ultimately to get the post you really want. It's likely that you'll maintain your links with your research group even while doing clinical work and this will have a positive impact on your approach to your patients. You will have gained new skills even in the most subspecialised PhD you can apply to everyday clinical practice. You will be a better doctor.

Key points

- You now know more about your topic than anyone else, but you need communicate this to others and spread what you have found to as wide an audience as possible.
- Publish, publish, publish! Cite your own work in letters, abstracts and papers. Attend meetings and conferences and present all your efforts.

Funding

9

Alex Clarke

■ Importance of funding

Research is expensive, and *you* are often the most expensive component. It is not surprising therefore that obtaining funding for your project is one of the biggest challenges in getting the research off the ground. Moreover funding becomes increasingly important as your academic career progresses, and many people may come to depend on your ability to convince a funding body that you and your research are worthy of their support. Funding is competitive, with application success rates for major clinical fellowships below 30%. This means that very often considerable resilience, perseverance and flexibility are required in the face of disappointment. Very few people in their academic careers will get every grant they apply for, and rejection at some stage is inevitable. That said, the funding is there for you to win and, as in any competition, there are many things you can do to improve your chances. Irrespective of your CV, awareness of potential funding sources, some of which may be off the beaten track, and persuasive grant writing are of paramount importance.

■ Understanding the funding process

At the forefront of your mind when planning your research should be the question: 'how will this project be paid for?' Fundamentally, you will either be applying for a pre-funded project, or need to bring the funding yourself via a research training or more senior fellowship or other personal grant. The former is usually more straightforward and quicker than the latter, but often comes with important strings attached. These may include limited ancillary funds for travel, conferences and course fees, and there could be significant clinical commitments, verging on the onerous. Pre-funded projects are often advertised in *BMJ Careers* or via the institution's own website.

Some departments will partially fund a project (often with so-called 'soft money') usually for 1 year, with the aim that some preliminary research will make a personal fellowship easier to win. Alternatively smaller grants may cover this period. Of course, if you can't get on-going funding the risk is that you will have spent a year with little to show for it.

Another important consideration is the timescale. It can take an inordinately long time from submission of the grant proposal to a decision (typically 6 months) and because you may not succeed at first, the process can run to 2 years. It's therefore crucial that you plan very early.

■ Important funding institutions and charities

There are hundreds of charities, governmental institutions, and commercial organisations that are potential sources of funding, although their pockets are of course hit by inclement economic times. Whilst it's impossible to cover all of these in detail, the major players are discussed in this chapter: the MRC, NIHR and the Wellcome Trust. An excellent place to start looking for funding opportunities is the NIHR-sponsored RD funding website (www.rdfunding.org.uk), which provides a comprehensive and up-to-the-minute searchable database.

The UK Government funds biomedical research through two main organisations: the MRC for basic medical science, and the NIHR for clinical projects. Charitable funding may be generic in the case of the Wellcome Trust, or disease specific, for example Cancer Research UK or the British Heart Foundation. Although the MRC, NIHR and Wellcome Trust may fund a variety of research, they do have specific 'themes' they consider to be deserving of special attention, and it is well worth considering these when writing your grant application. Research not meeting their aims will not be funded.

Medical Research Council

The Medical Research Council's (MRC's) major scheme for medical graduates leading to the award of a PhD, is the clinical research training fellowship (CRTF). To be eligible you must be in training (i.e. StR or below), and have completed the MRCP diploma or equivalent depending on clinical speciality. If you are an MB PhD graduate, you can still apply, as long as you haven't recently been active in research. Equally, if you have started a PhD (perhaps with 'soft money') you can also apply, as long as you have not been registered for more than 1 year. The MRC will allow you to spend two sessions a week (or three if you are a surgeon) on clinical duties. There are two opportunities to apply per year. The success rate for applications to the CRTF is around 30%. The MRC also co-sponsors (with a charity or Royal College) a number of disease area specific CRTFs, which are similar in detail to their general scheme. Information on these is available at their website (mrc.ac.uk).

National Institute for Health Research

The Doctoral Research Fellowship is the principal scheme for doctors of the NIHR. The NIHR is funded by the Department of Health and therefore as you might expect demands that applicants propose a project that 'demonstrates a role in, or contribution to, improving health care or services'. This means that the project has to be clinical research, and they stipulate that it must have the potential to impact upon patients within 5 years. They specifically won't fund research involving non-human tissue. Applications are accepted three times per year.

Wellcome Trust

The Wellcome Trust is the largest charity funding medical research and has two major schemes for medical graduates: the Research Training Fellowship (RTF) and the Clinical PhD Scheme. The RTF has a similar remit to the MRC's CRTF, and eligibility criteria are much the same. The Clinical PhD Scheme is unique to the Wellcome Trust however, and is a programme that funds the applicant to do research at a specific university/institution (currently Oxford, Cambridge, Imperial College London, Edinburgh, Dundee, Liverpool, and the London School of Hygiene and Tropical Medicine). The funding goes directly to the host unit, who then choose whom to recruit. The candidate does not need to have chosen a particular project at the time of application. Applications for the RTF are accepted three times each year, and the Clinical PhD varies depending on the host institution.

Other funding sources

There are many smaller charities that fund disease-specific research and smaller numbers of RTFs, so of course these are relevant to you and will depend on your project. A good place to find links to these charities is at the Association of Medical Research Charities website (amrc.org.uk) or the specialist society of your clinical speciality (e.g. the UK Renal Association or British Association of Dermatology).

What's funded?

This obviously varies according to the funding source but for fellowship schemes will generally include your personal salary, and up to a typical figure of £15 000 per year to cover consumables and attendance of conferences/travel. Typical fellowship schemes will not cover lab equipment and infrastructure costs, so your host institution must be fully equipped for your project. PhD fees may (e.g. MRC) or may not (e.g. Wellcome) be covered if your host institution does not waive them these can be substantial (£3000 per year). The personal salary paid will be your basic clinical salary (unbanded), dependent on seniority, and follows the standard NHS payscale. There may be some exceptions to this rule for pre-funded research.

▪ Applying for funding

Once you and your supervisor have identified an appropriate funding body and carefully studied their rules and deadlines, you will need to write a compelling grant application. This will require significant input from your research supervisor. Whilst the micromanagers amongst them may write the whole thing others may leave much more up to you. However, given that you will need in-depth knowledge of experimental techniques and often current unpublished research results, writing the whole application alone is not recommended. You should book time to sit with your supervisor to discuss your research project, formulate a research plan and design the experiments to test your hypotheses. You will need to perform a detailed literature review of your subject area to understand how your research fits into what is known. Your grant proposal must be edited to perfection and written in appropriate scientific style and you should ensure your supervisor critiques each draft, which can be a rate-limiting step.

Take the time to understand the facilities you have at your research institution and learn something about the techniques as you will be quizzed about this at interview. Know any controversies that surround your field of research. In order to write such a proposal it is highly beneficial to read previous grant proposals, particularly if others in the research group have done something similar.

Key points
- Applying for funding takes a lot of time – months to years! Start early
- Read the rules and regulations of your funding body
- Watch out for deadlines
- Thoroughly research the literature
- Read other grant proposals to understand the writing style required
- Think carefully about how you will conduct the study
- Learn about techniques you might use
- Involve the finance department of your research institution and the research governance office

If the proposed research involves human participation and/or animal work then the correct approvals need to be in place or in the process of being awarded. For all human work ethical approval is mandatory before any data can be collected. In animal research, a project license is required and you will need a personal Home Office license. This takes time!

The time it takes from settling on your project to the final application submission should not be underestimated, and may run from 6 months to 2 years, even without the need for preliminary data. It is absolutely vital to inform the training programme director for your clinical training scheme at the earliest opportunity, as you'll be leaving the rotation for a number of years and this has to be planned. Your deanery will also need advance notice, particularly if you intend to count your research towards your CCT.

Grant proposal

Your proposal will generally include:

* Abstract of the proposed investigation
  - Background
  - Aims
  - Methods
  - Main outcomes expected
* Lay summary
* Background of the project
  - Importance of question
  - What is not known
  - What you seek to investigate
* Original hypotheses
* Specific research objectives
* Experimental design of proposed investigation
  - Design
  - Population
  - Exposures
  - Follow up for outcomes
  - Key methodology
  - Statistical analysis
  - Data quality and management
  - Sample size
  - Ethics and research governance
* Expected value of results
* Scientific value
  - Your role on these studies
  - Formal research training
  - Career plans
  - Research training environment
* References.

A winning grant must contain evidence that you are worth funding, that the project is novel and will produce good results, and that the host laboratory is a suitable environment for the project, with a track record of supervision. These are the often quoted '**three Ps**' – **person, project, place**; and many application forms will explore each of these in a structured way.

Key points

* Be sure your project has a coherent direction and relevance for the future. This 'so what' of the research should run through the application as funders will want to see their money lead to real and measurable change

- Keep the sections of the plan well coordinated and clearly related to the central idea – every word must count
- Emphasise mechanism and scientific application but don't be overly ambitious – your plan should be based on a feasible timetable. Your specific aims and experiments should relate directly to the hypothesis to be tested

It's usually good advice when applying for anything to pay close attention to the assessment criteria, and most funding bodies publish these. Make sure that your application appropriately addresses each of them. This is often easier said than done in what may seem a severely limited space of a few thousand words. Assessors are generally looking for evidence that the project is of high scientific merit and will advance the organisation's research objectives, has a coherent and appropriate methodology, will provide the training required to advance in a scientific career, and that all this is achievable in the specified timescale.

The method by which you apply depends of course on the individual scheme, but there is a trend towards online forms that can be edited by several parties. This is much more convenient than emailing around a word-processed file and scanning signatures. Most application forms will cover your academic history and provide you an opportunity to demonstrate that you're the right person for the research project. You should detail your previous experience in research and explain exactly what you did. Your BSc project will be essential here. If you have none, collecting pilot data will support the application as well as demonstrating that you are suitable for the project. Your supervisor can assess your skills and this is important because your supervisor will need to make a statement about your suitability for the project. Adding a few figures is strongly recommended, for example a simple figurative representation of your project and any preliminary data, or of the timeline and planned 'milestones'.

You will have little expertise of budgeting, and you are unlikely to have much input in the finance part of the grant application, which can be very complex. Your supervisor and the departmental accountant or finance officer will do detailed costings for each part of your project, including your salary. Make sure they get it right! Your research equipment costs, computing costs, university fees and overheads will have been costed and included in your grant. They will also have considered your salary incremental dates – so that your salary rises year on year – and your superannuation (pension contributions).

Review of grant application

Your grant application will be reviewed in detail by two to six reviewers instructed by the funding body and you will receive their comments. This will provide guidance on the strengths and weaknesses of the application. They will assess the intellectual quality and potential impact of the study. Is it novel, and is it likely to succeed and produce new data? They will assess whether you have looked at the literature in enough detail, and presented evidence that might help to support your assertion that your hypothesis might be valid. They will also want the aims to be logical and interconnected, and the ensuing research procedures to be appropriate, adequate, and feasible for the research. They will want to know you have a suitable skills base, and that your planned supervisor and department are adequate and conducive to the research. If your grant proposal is considered worthy by your funding body, you are likely to be called to a competitive interview.

Interviews

The interview may occur up to 6 months after the initial submission. The nature of these vary but tend to include a large panel, perhaps more than 10 academics, of whom only a limited number will ask questions; the rest observe and score. Many interviews ask for a brief 'scene setting' presentation of a few minutes, either orally or using PowerPoint. The interview will then focus on your project, your knowledge of the research area and the science behind your project. They will also address contingencies such as what you would do if parts of the project failed to work. They will also seek your response to the reviewer's comments. You will need to defend your proposals and modify them according to the comments. Look at each and be sure to respond to each one. Be aware of your project's potential shortcomings, and prepare a robust defence for what may be quite intensive questioning.

> **Key points**
> * Know your proposals
> * Anticipate the questions
> * Fully prepare your answers to the reviewer's comments
> * Practise, practise, practise

Having direct experience of the experiments underlying your project can be invaluable here, and even if you haven't done substantive research at your proposed laboratory yet, it's strongly advisable to spend as much time as possible getting hands-on time with the equipment you'll be using. It's not unknown for interviewers to ask questions like 'so tell me how you do X', so be prepared.

The interview will also find out whether you have the ability, enthusiasm and motivation to succeed at PhD level. At the interview you are likely to be asked about your previous research experience (e.g. your BSc), your drive behind the planned PhD, as well as what you might intend to do after you have completed the PhD. They may also ask you how you will cope with the inevitable setbacks during your research, and your ability to deal with pressure and deadlines.

The interview itself can be a very stressful experience. The panel can appear intimidating and they may have read your prior publications and grill you on your past experience. They will expect clear and concise responses. Long rambling answers demonstrate that you cannot focus. It's highly recommended that you have mock interviews with your supervisor and other members of the department. It is more beneficial to have people with prior experience of grant funding bodies on the mock interview panel.

Clinical commitments during research

Your clinical commitments will vary according to the nature of your project, and with the funding source. The MRC and Wellcome Trust restrict the maximum number of clinical sessions to two per week. Other projects, particularly pre-funded ones, may ask for a lot more. The key question to ask is whether the proposed clinical duties will be excessive, and if they will enhance or detract from your research. Even two sessions per week will substantially reduce your research time, even if it does not sound much. Being on an on-call rota might be less intrusive as long as it does not take up daytime hours or leave you sleep deprived.

Unfortunately because it's more than likely you will be taking a pay cut (as your on-call supplement is lost during your research), you may need to top-up your income with locum work or as a body on an on-call rota. It is tempting to do too many locums or clinical work but of course there is the risk that you will end up tired and distracted; in all things, moderation! If you are lucky enough to get funding for your project, it may be worth letting the medical staffing department of your current hospital know that you will be available for locum work, as it will always be easier to be in a familiar environment. The major imperative though is the research: 3 years will fly by.

Insight into an academic's life

10

Ethics and research

Gavin W Sewell
Thean Soon Chew

A crucial part of any research you perform during your academic career will be governed by ethical considerations. Although ethical approval is essential for the research process it is often approached with a sense of dread, with the fear of drowning in a sea of paperwork. Like it or not, ethical approval is a crucial obstacle to negotiate before you can even begin your research, but is of course both critical for ensuring the highest standards of research and can also improve the research project. This chapter will aim to explain and demystify the processes involved in obtaining ethical approval. You should not have to cope with all of this alone when starting out in academia, and much will be done with the support of (or by) your supervisor.

▪ Why are ethics so important?

A fundamental requirement of any research study involving human subjects or animals is that it is carried out in accordance with current ethical principles. After the exploitation of vulnerable patients in the late nineteenth and early twentieth century, especially under the Nazi experimentation regime, there emerged a clear need for a consensual ethical framework for research studies. Many of the current principles are stated in the internationally recognised Declaration of Helsinki, which was first adopted by the World Medical Association (WMA) in 1964. There have since been six revisions, with the most current version being available on the WMA website (www.wma.net).

Some of the key principles established by the Declaration of Helsinki include:

* The need to seek informed consent from research participants.
* To respect their privacy and dignity.
* To acknowledge that participation in any study should be entirely voluntary.
* To recognise that the interest of the individual should always prevail over other interests, such as that of science and society.

A further requirement is that the design, performance and ethical considerations of any study must be described in a protocol. Ethics committees must assess whether a proposed protocol is in accordance with the principles of the Declaration of Helsinki.

Whilst the principles of the Declaration will be self-explanatory to many, the vast numbers of ethics committees, forms and websites and applications involved in the process can seem daunting and bewildering.

Different types of ethical approval

The nature of the research study will determine whether ethical approval is needed, the types of approval required and the process to be followed.

Does my project need ethical approval?

The first point to consider is whether your project is a research study or an audit. The National Research Ethics Service (NRES) defines a research study as:

> *"One that attempts to derive generalisable new knowledge, including studies that aim to generate hypotheses as well as studies that aim to test them".*

In contrast, an audit is "designed to evaluate a service against a predetermined 'gold standard', which will inform current clinical practice and delivery of care". An audit never involves randomisation of subjects and usually involves analysis of existing data. However, research may involve randomisation of subjects into groups and usually involves collection of data additional to those for routine care.

If your project is a research study, then you will need to apply for ethical approval, and if the study is taking place within the NHS, then review by an NRES committee is necessary. On the other hand, if your project is an audit or service evaluation, ethical approval is not required – and you may breathe a sigh of relief!

My project is a research study involving NHS patients. What approval do I need?

If your research study involves NHS patients, you should submit an application to an NRES committee, who will assess whether it conforms to current ethical guidelines. The first step is setting up an account on the Integrated Research and Application System (IRAS) website (www.myresearchproject.org.uk), completing the application form and submitting it to your local Regional Ethics Committee (REC) or centrally via the Central Allocation System. You will also need research and development (R&D) approval at sites where the research is being carried out; the forms for this can be generated on the IRAS website. Each NHS Trust will have a R&D office to assist in this process, and advise what forms need to be completed.

> ### Useful information
>
> Ethical review from a NHS research ethics committee is required for any research involving the following:
> - Patients (past or present) treated within the NHS, and even patients treated under contracts with private sector institutions
> - Relatives or carers of other NHS patients who have been identified as potential research participants
> - When access is needed to data, organs, or other bodily material of NHS patients (past or present)
> - Fetal material and in vitro fertilisation involving NHS patients
> - Patients who have died recently within NHS institutions
> - When using NHS facilities or properties
> - Recruitment of NHS staff as potential research participants by virtue of their professional role
> - Recruitment of healthy volunteers, if performed on NHS premises

Special circumstances

If your study is a clinical trial involving administration of a drug (otherwise known as an 'investigative medicinal product'), then you will also need Medicines and Healthcare products Regulatory Agency (MHRA) approval before you commence the trial. However, certain substances are exempt from this, including human whole blood and plasma, food products such as dietary supplements, as well as surgical interventions.

> ### Key point
>
> For clinical trials involving administration of a drug, you should check the MHRA website (www.mhra.gov.uk) for up-to-date requirements. The MHRA application forms can be downloaded and completed on the IRAS website.

For such a study, you will need to submit an application form, clinical trial protocol, a brochure or dossier giving information about the drug, certification of good manufacturing practice and ethics committee approval once this is available.

> ### Beware!
>
> - Fees charged by the MHRA are not insignificant. Currently it costs more than £4000 for approval of a Phase II patient trial and more than £2000 for a Phase I healthy volunteer trial. Ensure you have budgeted for this in your trial costs/sponsorship.

Additional approvals may be needed for research involving administration of:

* Radioactive substances.

* Gene and stem cell therapy.
* Medical devices and research involving human gametes and embryos.

You will need to send an additional application form to the relevant committee, some of which can be generated in the IRAS website.

What if my research study involves human subjects but not NHS patients?

If your study involves human subjects, but not NHS patients, their relatives or NHS staff, then you would normally submit an application to an ethics committee specific to your university or institution. These committees may be made up of university academics, lay members, clinicians and pharmacists. The precise nature of the application may vary slightly between institutions, but will usually require submission of project and sponsor details, a project protocol, participant information sheets and consent forms, and a risk assessment. Exceptions to the rule in this situation include research involving prisoners and individuals lacking capacity to consent, in which case an application must be made to an NRES committee for ethical approval.

■ Understanding ethics committees and the process

The first step in applying for ethical approval is creating an online account on the IRAS website. This website allows you to generate application forms for a number of different types of approval using the same project dataset, including ethics, MHRA and research and development, so (in theory) saving time, unnecessary duplication and form filling!

Beware!

The online forms can be challenging at times – try not to become disheartened and remember to ask for help if you are struggling!

After completing the online application form you are ready to book a 'slot' for ethical review – your local R&D office will explain how to do this. If you are conducting a clinical trial, you should contact the Central Allocation System, who will arrange for an appropriate REC to review the study (which may not be the REC at the trial site). In most other situations, you can contact your local REC directly to book a slot. A list of RECs, together with meeting dates, is published on the NRES website (www.nres.npsa.nhs.uk).

Key point

Ensure you submit your applications at least 14 days prior to the REC meetings to avoid any delays with your applications.

Once you have a confirmed slot with a REC, you should send them hard signed copies of all documents. After submission, an ethical opinion on the study must be given by the REC within 60 days, although in practice most committees communicate their decisions sooner than this. You should factor this time into any research plans.

An ethics committee typically consists of:

* Doctors.
* Nurses.
* Pharmacists.
* Statisticians.
* Lay members (who make up approximately one-third of the committee).

Some members may have specialist experience in ethics, philosophy or theology. The committee may sometimes invite applicants to the meeting. Attendance is advisable as discussion between the applicant and committee may help clarify and resolve any concerns or queries that are raised.

At the meeting, the committee will agree their final decision. This can be one of four outcomes:

1 Approval (where no further amendments are needed).
2 Conditional approval (minor alterations required, but without re-review).
3 Provisional approval (where more substantial changes may be needed, and re-review by a subcommittee).
4 Rejection.

Less than 20% of studies are approved with no amendments, although very few applications are rejected outright. A letter detailing the decision is usually sent to the applicant within 10 working days.

Typical requirements for ethical approval of studies involving human subjects

---

Useful information

Ordinarily you will need to submit the following:
* IRAS application form
* Research protocol (including explanation in lay terms)
* Participant information sheets
* Consent forms
* Curriculum vitae from investigators
* Details of indemnity arrangements
* Sponsors details

In addition, it may be helpful to include a covering letter and any relevant letters from sponsors, referees or statisticians.

The ethics committee will assess the significance of the research and whether the potential risks of the study outweigh the benefits. Note that the ethics committee will not assess the scientific quality of the research per se; this is the role of the project sponsor, although the committee will need evidence that the project has been subject to a rigorous scientific review.

The committee will also play close attention to the patient information sheets and consent forms; these are often the areas that let down an application and need amendment. Get your non-medical mother to read them!:

* **Information sheet** – This should provide the participant with a clear, concise summary of the background to the study, and the potential benefits and risks. The language should be easily comprehensible to a lay person; medical and scientific jargon should be avoided. You should also describe how you are going to protect their personal data and maintain confidentiality, and how you are going to report your findings back to the participants at the end of the study (see Smajdor *et al*, in Further Reading). It is certainly helpful to stick to a generic format and some useful suggestions and templates can be found on the NRES website. It may be useful to have different information sheets for different study groups. They may also need to be available in languages other than English.
* **Consent form** – If your study involves several different groups of patients, or indeed patients and control volunteers, then it may be helpful to create separate consent forms for each group in a similar way to the information sheets. In addition, if your study involves individuals younger than 18 years of age you will need to create specific consent forms for these patients. Consent forms for patients aged less than 5 years should be mostly pictorial.

The provisions for maintaining confidentiality, as well as long-term storage of patient samples and data, will be assessed by the committee. It helps to give specific details such as who will have access, where will it be stored and for how long (e.g. information will be stored within an encrypted database on a password-protected computer located in a secure department).

Ethics for animal studies

Animal experimentation is a highly emotive subject both inside and outside of the research world. You will have a personal view on the ethical position. Without question, research performed on animals has allowed many major advances within the medical and scientific world. However, before you start considering research involving animals you must consider very carefully the ethics of animal research. It is a highly regulated process that must be adhered too without exception – not only for ethical reasons, but also as there are strict laws related to this work and failure to adhere can lead to prosecution. On research ethics application forms you will need to fill in additional details.

When considering animal research you must consider 'the 3Rs':

* Replacement.

* Reduction.
* Refinement.

This approach is based on the programme of the National Centre for the Replacement, Reduction and Refinement in Animal Research, which was established by the UK Government and funded by the Wellcome Trust, Medical Research Council (MRC) and Biotechnology and Biological Sciences Research Council (BBSRC) to support science, innovation and animal welfare in bioscience:

* **Replacement** – You need to consider if your research question can be answered without the use of animals before you start a project. Whilst animals can provide a useful biological system to test the safety of drugs and create models of disease, can the same research question be better answered by *replacing* animals with computational models, cell lines, in vitro techniques or even humans?
* **Reduction** – If animal research is essential, then consider if *reducing* the number of animals is possible to obtain the same amount of information or if more information could be obtained from the fixed minimum number of animals you have to use.
* **Refinement** – You must ensure you *refine* your research so to minimise the harm, suffering and pain endured by the animals by setting severity limits, using analgesia, and ensuring enrichment of life for the animals.

Your supervisor would have already considered these issues, and you cannot conduct animal research without significant support, but it is an important part of your long-term training as a researcher to consider these issues carefully.

Animal research and the Law

The Animals (Scientific Procedures) Act 1986 and the European Union (EU) Directive 86/609 mainly govern animal research in the UK. Knowing the laws that govern animal research in the UK are your responsibility as a researcher using animals. However, do not be put off animal research by the Law since it may help answer fundamental questions! The Law is there to protect and maintain standards of care of laboratory animals. If you will be working with animals, your host institution will almost always have a taught course on animal care which you will have to attend.

Useful information

Animal welfare law in the United Kingdom existed before laws that protected children from cruelty. In 1822, 2 years before the Royal Society for the Prevention of Cruelty to Animals (RSPCA) was formed, Martin's Act was passed that forbade the cruel treatment of cattle. However, only in 1889 was the Prevention of Cruelty to Children Act passed, after lobbying by Reverend Benjamin Waugh, founder of the National Society for the Prevention of Cruelty to Children (NSPCC).

Depending on the exact nature of your research, other laws may also be relevant, for example the Medicines Act 1966 if you are administering controlled drugs. The Animals (Scientific Procedures) Act 1986 defines what a protected animal is, what constitutes living or dead, mandates the standard methods of killing and a list of animals that can only come from designated suppliers. The Act contains a three-fold licensing system:

1 **Certificate of designation** – This determines physical locations where scientific procedures can be carried out, species to be housed and conditions. The certificate also designates a Certificate Holder (someone who is in charge overall), a Named Veterinary Surgeon (NVS) and a Named Animal Care & Welfare Officer (NACWO). This is the responsibility of the staff at your university's animal unit.

2 **A project license** – This outlines the experiments that can be performed, the species of animals and places permitted for work. There will usually be a project license under the name of your research supervisor/principal investigator or the Head of Department for the department you work in. The project licensee is responsible for the direction, compliance, training and supervision of personal licensees under the project.

3 **A personal license** – It is your responsibility to obtain a personal license. Without it, you *cannot* perform any procedures on animals. As soon as you are sure you will be involved with animal research you must book to attend an animal license course and identify the species that you will be working with, i.e. mouse, rat, gerbil, rabbit, fish, etc. Most large universities will run certified animal license courses that are accredited by either the Institute of Biology, Universities' Accreditation Scheme or the Scottish Accreditation Board. There is a set curriculum issued by the Home Office.

Beware!

You do not automatically pass this test! You can fail and then lose the money for the cost of the course! Prepare well in advance.

Once you have passed the test, you will be issued with a certificate. You will then need to download and fill in the personal license application form from the Home Office website (www.homeoffice.gov.uk/science-research/animal-research). You will be asked to list all the procedures that you will need for your experiments from a list of specified procedures in the guidance notes. The Home Office then issues a *personal license* for you to perform the set list of procedures under a specified *project license* at the *designated* site. Your supervisor will usually pay for the course and license from their grants, but do check with them.

The Animals (Scientific Procedures) Act 1986 requires that you, the *personal license holder*, abide by the Act and only perform the specified procedures on the specified animals at the specified places. There is a list of 22 standard conditions on the license that you need to abide by. Any contravention of the Act will result in an initial written warning, retraining, withdrawal of the license, a fine or ultimately imprisonment.

> **Key points**
>
> When considering animal research:
>
> 1 Determine how much of your research will involve animals and what species.
> 2 Always consider your own ethical position on animal research – be aware of what it involves early on.
> 3 Book an animal license course as soon as possible – it is essential before you can get ethical approval.
> 4 Understand what samples you need from the animals.
> 5 Apply for the license early and list the required procedures you will be undertaking.

Overcoming setbacks

Applying for ethics can be a drawn-out, frustrating process at times! Don't be surprised or disheartened if you need to make changes to your application before it gets approved. In addition to their decision, the Committee will provide you with feedback and details of changes required. Think about these carefully before re-submitting the application again:

* What were their main concerns? For example, was the patient information sheet too vague or too complex? This is a common problem.
* Were there problems with the protocol itself? Speak to your supervisors and colleagues, and seek advice from others who have made ethics applications in the past.

If possible, apply and obtain ethical approval before you start in your clinical academic research position. Otherwise it is possible to waste a lot of time at the beginning just sending applications back and forth to ethics committees! If you really can't apply for ethics before you start, begin some back-up or side projects that already have approval or do not require it while the application is being processed – so if it is rejected then you aren't left without any projects to work on!

Alterations to pre-existing research

Amendments

Sometimes, a research study will need to be adjusted or altered after ethical approval has been obtained. Such 'amendments' are classified as either substantial or non-substantial.

Substantial amendments

These are alterations that may affect the safety of the subjects in the study, the conduct or management of the study or its scientific value. Examples include changes to procedures undertaken by participants (such as taking an additional blood sample), major changes to patient information sheets, or a change of chief investigator. The main REC should be notified of any substantial amendments, and for clinical trials, documentation should be submitted to the MHRA. You should complete a 'Notice of Substantial Amendment' form detailing the change(s) and reasons for it. This form can be generated in the IRAS website, or alternatively you can obtain a copy from your local REC. With your application, you should also include copies of any altered documentation (such as patient information sheets), highlighting the key changes. If it is valid, the notice of substantial amendment will be reviewed by a REC sub-committee and a decision communicated to you within 35 days.

Non-substantial amendments

These are alterations that you do not need to notify the main REC about. Sponsors or chief investigators still wishing to do so should merely write a covering letter to the committee explaining that amendments are not substantial and ethical opinion is not necessary. Examples include typographical errors, changes in funding arrangements etc.

Site-specific approval

You may find that during the course of your project you need to involve other hospitals or sites in addition to the main one. This could be to help recruit additional patients to a clinical trial, or to obtain additional tissue samples for a laboratory-based study. You do not need to make separate ethics applications for each site providing that the protocol is the same. You should, however, obtain the approval of the R&D office at that proposed site. You should fill out the 'Site-specific Approval' application on the IRAS website, and send it, together with other relevant documentation, to the appropriate office.

Key points

When applying for ethical approval for research:

- Apply early – it takes time
- Try not to lose heart – you will get there in the end
- If you are not sure about something – ask for help!
- Ask for help and guidance anyway!
- Keep your options open – if your application is rejected make sure you have a back-up plan
- Remember special considerations with animal research
- Be nice to your local Research and Development office!

Further reading

UK Integrated Research Application System. www.myresearchproject.org.uk

National Centre for the Replacement, Refinement and Reduction of Animals in Research (2010) *What are the 3Rs?* Available at: www.nc3rs.org.uk

National Research Ethics Service (NRES) documentation. www.nres.npsa.nhs.uk

Smajdor A, Sydes MR, Gelling L, Wilkinson M. Applying for ethical approval for research in the United Kingdom. *BMJ* 2009;339:4013

Vollman J, Winau R. Informed consent in human experimentation before the Nuremberg code. *BMJ* 1996;313:1445–7

World Medical Association. www.wma.net

11

Publications and presentations

Daniel JB Marks
Philip J Smith

A fundamental aspect of academia is the communication of research findings to other scientists and clinicians. Writing for publication is both exciting and daunting. Papers change practice, and a particularly salient article can be downloaded and read by several thousand researchers. That said, the road to publication can at times be long and frustrating, with numerous obstacles along the way. Your manuscript may require several revisions before it is finally accepted.

Presentations at meetings and conferences also assist in the distribution of your data and stimulate open debate in the research community. Do not underestimate the time required to prepare a strong oral or poster presentation – much thought and effort are required.

What should be published?

To date, over 50 million scientific papers have been published, there are approximately 20 000 scientific journals, and over 5000 new articles are published daily. Sadly, a subculture has emerged of writing for the primary purpose of obtaining publications, rather than to share important scientific results. This was perhaps best expressed by Richard Asher, writing in the *British Medical Journal* in 1958:

> "If a man has something to say which interests him, and he knows how to say it, then he need never be dull. Some people have a desire for publication but nothing more. They have nothing to say, and do not know how to say it. They want to be seen in the British Medical Journal or the Lancet because it is respectable to be seen there. They would stand no chance of publication

in lay magazines, but the number of medical journals is so large that
every dog has his day." Asher R. Why are medical journals so dull?
BMJ 1958;2:502–3

For a paper to be publishable, it must be original, relevant and scientifically
valid. It should also be clear and well written, but whilst poor English language
can be corrected during the review and editing process, the three principle
tenets cannot:

1 **Novelty** – If your research is only marginally different to that already
   available, there must be something in particular that justifies its publication.
   This could include extending the study to a new population, intervention, or
   outcome measure. There must, however, be a plausible argument that this
   variation could produce different results.
2 **Relevance** – There is no point answering a question that nobody is asking.
   The paper should either add significantly to knowledge in areas of current
   interest or open new avenues for investigation.
3 **Validity** – There must be a clear and logical progression from the research
   question to the conclusion. The question must be clearly defined, the
   answer not known *a priori*, and the problem must be intrinsically soluble.
   Most importantly, can the methods employed produce results that reliably
   answer the question posed, and are the conclusions drawn justifiable?
   To assess validity, expect reviewers to scrutinise your Methods section
   in depth.

Different types of publications

Clinical trials and original scientific articles

Clinical trials and original scientific articles are the most sought-after
publications within the science world. Scientific articles describe in detail the
results of original research findings, and play a very important role. They can
often change opinion on the pathogenesis of disease, the understanding of
previously accepted theories and the direction of future research. Similarly,
a well-designed randomised–controlled clinical trial can change the face of
clinical practice.

Be aware that formal randomised clinical trials now often need to be
registered with a central monitoring body prior to commencement. In Europe,
this is an absolute requirement for trials sponsored by the pharmaceutical
industry. This was originally intended to increase awareness of non-publication
of studies with negative results to try and reduce publication bias when
systematically reviewing the evidence base. It also allows reviewers and readers
the facility to check whether research has been performed and presented in the
way that was originally planned, rather than in a manner that encourages sales
of a drug. In particular, they can ensure that the reported primary outcomes

and analyses are those that were originally intended, not those that *post hoc* have been found to deliver 'preferable' findings.

> **Beware!**
>
> From the point of view of publication, many journals will exclude trials that are not appropriately registered. If in doubt, register!

Reviews and meta-analyses

Both of these types of publications are commonplace within the scientific literature. The authors do not describe their own original scientific research, but instead accumulate the results from many different studies or trials on a particular topic, and assimilate this into an important narrative and overview on the current understanding on that subject. Review articles act as a source of information and reference on a particular topic, whereas meta-analyses provide quantitative estimates from multiple studies to help understand and test certain hypotheses. There are clearly defined methods for conducting meta-analyses or systematic reviews, for example from the Cochrane Collaboration.

Letters

Academic letters published within journals are short descriptions of important current research findings, or expert opinions on previously published articles or reviews. They are often published fairly rapidly because they are considered important for stimulating debate in academic circles and can add additional context to research findings.

Case reports

Case reports are sometimes dismissed as unimportant publications, as critics describe them as being of 'little scientific interest' since they provide no evidence base. Nonetheless, many believe they fulfil several important roles. Firstly, they may highlight a new clinical presentation or management technique; subsequent case reports amalgamate into series, and thus a new clinical entity or treatment is born. Indeed, some journals have identified case reports amongst their most cited articles. Secondly they educate, highlighting cases of interest with particular learning points to colleagues and stimulating recognition or recollection, even if previously described. Finally, they are often entertaining, providing a welcome interlude from an otherwise dry scientific journal.

> **Beware!**
>
> Beware when submitting a report that includes a disproportionate number of authors for a straightforward case as this will be viewed with suspicion. Having seen the patient once on a ward round or booking an investigation does not qualify for authorship!

Writing style

There are no fixed rules regarding writing style, but there are a few important principles. Whatever your personal style, you should adapt it in accordance with the journal recommendations, and follow their requirements meticulously. Aim for brevity and simplicity of writing; avoid being pretentious. Unclear writing indicates that your ideas are not yet well developed. Your aim is to assist the reader and guide them through your work and thought processes. Ensure that each sentence is on topic and entirely relevant, that the relationship between sentences is clear and logical, and that the main ideas are communicated and supported by specific evidence. Clarity is ultimately what matters most, and this is largely a matter of time and effort. Jargon and abbreviations should be avoided where possible.

Reviewers or editors will not generally alter a particular author's style, but usually expect correct grammar, spelling and punctuation. Isolated and infrequent typographic mistakes are generally overlooked in submitted papers and corrected by subeditors, but if recurrent are particularly irritating, especially when they impede readability. Greater leniency is often afforded to non-English speakers. Inaccuracies can be reduced by careful proofreading prior to submission, but it is well-recognised that having written multiple drafts, authors become increasingly familiar with the paper and fail to spot simple errors. Ask colleagues to help.

There has been considerable debate as to the use of the active (as opposed to the passive) voice, and fashions change over time. Whilst the active was originally favoured in publications, about 3 decades ago the third person passive gained preference as it was seen as more detached and objective. There has now been a swing back towards the first person active, which is felt to be clearer. Similarly, the present tense is generally preferred. Use whichever produces the most readable text.

In scientific writing, brevity is a virtue! Most journals will set a limit of 3500–4000 words; this will be indicated in the 'Instructions to Authors'. If you exceed this, check that your results are not duplicated (including within the Tables and Figures), that your literature review is absolutely relevant and not overly excessive, and remove any tangential discussion. Medical articles should, like after-dinner speeches, finish before the audience's interest has started to wane.

Writing support

This typically involves the employment of a professional writer to assist in drafting of manuscripts. Modest support is not necessarily prohibited, and may improve the quality of the article. It should, however, always be acknowledged, as it will otherwise be considered 'ghost-writing', that is the persons taking credit for publication of the manuscript and the data therein are not those who actually wrote the paper. There has been increasing awareness of this as a problem over recent years, with the popular media having become aware of drug companies 'ghost-writing' under the guise of other scientists. Always review and abide by individual journal policies.

Key points

- Keep it succinct
- Avoid jargon and abbreviations as much as possible
- Read the 'Instructions to Authors' and follow the journal recommendations
- Proofread, proofread, proofread – and ask others to proofread too!

Structure of scientific papers

With the exception of narrative reviews, scientific papers are usually subdivided according to the Abstract, Introduction, Methods, Results and Discussion/Conclusion (IMRaD structure). A few journals are notable exceptions, such as *Nature* and *Science*. Case reports tend to have a Case Description in place of the Methods and Results. For general guidelines, see the International Committee of Medical Journal Editors (ICMJE, www.icmje.org). Always follow the journal's instructions carefully, particularly with regards to formatting of the manuscript and references. Failure to do so irritates both editors and reviewers, and may be seen as indicative of a general lack of attention to detail that can undermine your paper. If authors cannot be bothered to follow simple instructions, then they are perhaps also not bothered about adopting the meticulous approach needed to generate high-quality research.

Although there is a standardised structure to articles, and each section is described here in sequence, it is often most helpful to start write an article in the following order:

1 Create your tables and figures first. Your results are what your paper is trying to communicate, and in this way you can clarify the story you are going to elaborate.
2 Next write the Methods and Results, such that the order of the text follows that in which the data are presented.
3 Finally, write your Introduction and Discussion, so that they are totally relevant to your findings.

Authorship

Authorship is sadly a frequent source of discord with colleagues, both in terms of inclusion and sequence. It is important to realise that authorship commits you to the data presented, *for better or worse*, and means you have contributed materially to the paper. Many are attracted to the glory of the paper on the CV.

Few consider the ignominy of having a paper retracted, in which all authors share guilt by association. Generally speaking, the person who acquired the majority of the data and who writes the paper merits first authorship. Occasionally, when there has been close collaboration, it is appropriate to have joint first authorship, accompanied by a statement that both parties have contributed equally to the work. The sequence should then run according to the level of input. Senior authorship is typically reserved for the person with the greatest conceptual input into the study.

Title

It is worth spending some time perfecting your paper's title. It is the most prominent statement in the manuscript, and informs readers what information will be presented. It is particularly strongly represented in literature searches, and should be attractive but not sensationalised. Your title should be one that triages the manuscript to the appropriate readership. Try to use key words that resonate with the rest of the article, particularly its primary concepts and variables. Most titles either describe the research question ('An investigation into...') or the pertinent result ('Beta-blockers cause...'). Occasionally, for reviews and editorials, the title may instead indicate the author's position on a particular topic or ask a specific question.

Be concise, ideally using fewer than 12 words. Opinions are heated over the inclusion of punctuation, and this should be kept to a minimum. Colons are acceptable, particularly if they precede design elements of the study or research quality indicators such as 'a systematic review' or 'a retrospective study'. If posing a question, ensure your title does not sound trite when you read it.

Abstract

Many (possibly most) readers will only ever read the abstract! Particular care should be taken over this section of the paper, which is sometimes left as an afterthought. It is the only part universally accessible and searched through electronic databases. Since not all individuals or institutions have access to the full manuscript, readers will often draw conclusions from the abstract. It is therefore important to make sure that this is genuinely representative of the overall content of the paper. Be aware that most journals impose a word limit of approximately 250 words; exceeding this may result in the abstract being cropped when captured in some electronic databases.

Introduction

The introduction should be brief. It is there to provide the appropriate framework for the reader to understand the background to your paper. As such, there should be both a theoretical component outlining the problem area, as well as a summary of the empirical data currently available. It is not intended to be an in-depth literature review: its purpose is to explain the research question, why it is relevant and original, and very briefly how it will be approached.

Materials and methods

This section will be used primarily to assess the validity and reliability of your study. A statement must be made if relevant regarding ethical approval for the study (including the authority granting approval and a reference number), and how consent was obtained and recorded. The Methods should describe exactly how the study was performed, with sufficient information to allow the reader to reproduce the work. The sources of all reagents, assays and equipment should be cited, as there may be important variation between different manufacturers.

It is particularly important to describe the statistics accurately. This should include how summary statistics are presented (for example, averages as means or medians; ranges as standard deviations, standard errors or interquartile range). Some justification as to the numbers of subjects studied or observations performed is helpful, occasionally accompanied by a formal calculation of statistical power. Comparative studies should indicate the degree of difference regarded as being biologically or clinically of relevance, *prior* to commencing the study. *Post hoc* power calculations are of almost no value, and will be treated as such by reviewers.

Results

This section should start with a contextual description of whom or what was studied, indicating how many subjects were recruited or experiments were performed, and how many successfully completed the study. If relevant, consider summarising this in a patient flow diagram. All subjects should be accounted for, including those enrolled but not studied, those withdrawn and protocol violations. Traditionally demographic data are presented next. If groups are randomised, descriptive statistics and comparisons should be presented, although hypothesis testing should not be applied to randomised baseline data.

Main outcome data should be described in the text, with the primary outcomes before secondary. Figures and tables provide more detail. The text should highlight key data, but not duplicate those presented visually. Symmetrically distributed data should be summarised using the mean and standard deviation and analysed with parametric tests such as the students *t*-test. Skewed data should be expressed using the median and interquartile range, and analysed with non-parametric tests such as the Mann–Whitney *U*-test. Appropriate tests or corrections must be applied for multiple comparisons on the same data set. For important outcomes, raw data should be presented where possible. Continuously distributed outcome measures may be displayed by group using dot plots for smaller samples, or box and whisker diagrams for larger samples.

One area where reviewers may be particularly critical is with use of the P value and the concept of statistical significance. These are widely misinterpreted. Precision in this area is vital, as seemingly minor errors easily lead to unjustified conclusions and hence potentially incorrect clinical decisions. Reporting of results from multiple tests should be avoided wherever possible, as the more that are performed, the more likely 'evidence' will emerge by chance. You should plan exactly what single test will be performed on primary outcome before starting the study.

There are two important aspects to any observed difference between a study and control group: the magnitude of the difference, and the degree of uncertainty surrounding it. The magnitude of the difference may or may not be of clinical significance. For example, if studying the effect of a new antiviral drug for the treatment of glandular fever in a large number of patients, a symptomatic resolution that was 1 hour faster in the treatment as opposed to the control arm may be observed as statistically significant, but is of little importance in the context of the practical use of the drug.

The P value is often paraphrased as the probability that any observed difference was purely due to chance. It is important to be aware that the choice of $P=0.05$ as a threshold for significance is entirely arbitrary. It is misleading to use this as a benchmark of proof, and more helpful to interpret the P value as an indication of the strength of evidence. It is therefore advisable to report the absolute P value; that is, a P of 0.02 indicates stronger evidence than one of 0.05. This is much more helpful than stating $P<0.05$, as it helps the reader understand the possible level of error with your data. Extreme caution should be used with the word 'trend' when describing differences with a $P>0.05$; its use should be reserved for describing a pattern of data as function of another variable such as time or dose.

Confidence intervals are particularly helpful as they provide the reader with information on the range of values within which the true (as opposed to the measured sample) difference may actually lie. The 95% interval is usually chosen, although this is also arbitrary. At the end of the day, the interpretation of what is a clinically significant and important difference may be subjective. Presenting full data including confidence intervals allows clinicians to interpret the results for themselves, and decide whether to modify their own practice on the basis of your evidence.

Tables and figures

Tables and figures should be interpretable in isolation, and in general your work should be understandable from the data presented in diagrams, charts and tables. Take time to try different presentations and arrangements. For example, when constructing a graph, consider use of different axes and ordinates, hatching and shading. Diagrams should only be used if they make something easier to understand. Reviewers get particularly annoyed when the numbers in tables do not add up, or if there are inconsistencies between the text, tables and figures.

Discussion

There is no set format for the discussion. You should in general concentrate on the hard findings from the study, but can include subjective judgements about these. It is advisable to begin by stating the answer you have found to your research question, and how this ties in with the study aims. You should not repeat the results and introduction in details. Focus on the primary outcome, and include comments as to relevance of your findings. You should highlight how these are novel, but do not exaggerate. They also need to be placed in context, in particular how they relate to other available studies. If the latter are numerous, only the salient points need be included. If your results are different than expected, and the reasons for this are unclear, you may state as much. It is reasonable to speculate in your discussion, but be transparent that this is theoretical. Data may be genuinely inconsistent for good reasons, which may not yet be known, and providing your methodology is sound future work will clarify the situation. You should openly discuss the strengths and limitations of your studies, especially when compared with similar work. No study is perfect, and identifying areas of weakness adds to its credibility.

Conclusion

If a conclusion is included, this must be succinct (one or two sentences) restating how your findings answered the research question. Give a take-home message. Avoid ambiguous non-statements such as 'more work is needed/more studies need to be done'; they are weak and add nothing.

References

The references should be up to date, absolutely relevant and accurately support any statements made. Some references are likely to be written by people asked to review your paper; misquoting them does not help! Many referees will scrutinise and read key references, and will pounce on any inaccuracy. Each journal will have its own in-house style for the References section and citation within the text; see the Instructions for Authors for details. Use of programmes such as Reference Manager or Endnote is invaluable, particularly when revisions to the manuscript are required.

Acknowledgements

You should acknowledge all substantial assistance, especially financial. In the case of the latter, it is helpful to indicate the extent of involvement of any funding body in terms of study design, data collection and analyses, interpretation, writing of the manuscript and the decision for publication.

Acknowledge anyone who helped with data collection or interpretation not included in the authorship, as well as those who proofread your paper prior to submission.

Contributorship

More and more journals now require a statement of contributorship, outlining exactly what role each author played in the study. This is not only to ensure that authorship is justified, but provides appropriate accountability for the components of the work. For example, it may be unreasonable to expect a statistician to identify flaws in the methodology of a biological experiment, just as an immunologist may struggle to spot errors in a complex mathematical model. One author (usually the senior scientist on the paper) may be asked to be the guarantor for the article.

Conflicts of interest

These are usually interpreted to mean actions potentially taken to satisfy private interests that may not serve the best interests of the wider community. Journals do not assess the behaviour of authors relative to each specific submission, but publish disclosure statements so that readers are aware of any potential to bias. Common conflicts include equity interests, corporate relationships, patent rights, consultancies, family relationships and funding for research. Rarely there can be political or religious conflicts. When in doubt, declare! It will not jeopardise publication, but could be disastrous if an undeclared conflict is later judged to have unduly influenced the work.

Key points
- Consider authorship carefully
- Take time over the title: it is the 'headline grabber' but shouldn't be sensationalised
- Remember most people will only ever read the abstract – make it representative of the publication as a whole
- In your discussion, summarise your findings first, then place them in the context of other studies
- If you have a conflict of interest – declare it!
- Don't be tempted to publish 'too soon' – it may be by waiting a bit longer, and including more information, you have an even stronger paper
- Don't be tempted to divide your research into too many pieces – one excellent publication is better than a number of weaker ones

▪ Choosing a journal

You have worked hard to produce original research, now it is important to choose the best journal to send it to. There are a multitude of journals available to which you could potentially submit your article. Your principal consideration should be how to best disseminate your paper to those clinicians and scientists to whom it will be most relevant. Try to establish the readership of each journal. Look at what they have previously published and whether your article would fit in with these. It may be helpful to review the reference list from your own manuscript to see which journals crop up! Ask for advice from other experts in the field and your supervisors.

An area of much contention is the impact factor (IF) of a journal, which is based on the number of citations received by the average paper it publishes. Sadly, there can be a lot of intellectual snobbery around this. Whilst a publication in a high IF journal is certainly a cause for celebration, remember that there are plenty of excellent and important papers in other publications. In fact, the latter may be a better way to bring your data to the attention of researchers with a particular subspeciality interest. Further, many high IF journals will not publish research that is too specialised since it will not be relevant to a general readership.

Useful information

The impact factor (IF) of a journal is the ratio of the average number of citations to the total number of citable items that were published during the 2 preceding years. IFs are calculated yearly for journals that are listed in Journal Citation Reports (a report produced by Healthcare Division of Information company, Thomson Reuters).

Realistic expectations

It is very difficult when you have potentially been working on a piece of research for a significant period of time to maintain an objective perspective. However, occasionally you will recognise that your data are not of sufficient calibre to merit publication in a high IF journal. Nonetheless, it may still be valuable to submit to one of these first, as such journals often have better access to more experienced peer reviewers. Although rejecting the manuscript, their suggestions can considerably enhance its quality or highlight what additional work needs to be performed.

Peer review

Peer review is one way of ensuring the quality of a paper. Whilst good reviews improve papers immeasurably, the process is not always perfect and can at times be frustrating. There is no universal formula for the review process, and all have their own nuances and styles. Try to think like a reviewer when writing and critically proofread your manuscript, and address problem areas proactively rather than responsively.

Many journals invite authors to nominate potential reviewers, although they are not obliged to use your recommendations. You are looking for someone with sufficient experience and knowledge in the field to adequately critique your paper.

> ## Beware!
>
> Having to retract a flawed paper subsequent to its publication is a disaster. Remember that while it may be disappointing to get a negative review, it is far better than having to deal with the former!

If you are not personally familiar with other researchers in your field, seek guidance from senior colleagues. If this fails, a good starting point is your own reference list from the paper, to identify those who have recently published on a related issue. Similarly, be aware that some reviewers may (inappropriately) take it as a personal slight if you have not cited their work; diplomacy may be important with your selection! You can also sometimes request that individuals who you feel may have a personal or professional conflict of interest with your work are not nominated for the review process.

The rejected paper

The majority of manuscripts submitted for publication will initially be rejected at the editorial or peer-review stage. Do not lose heart – 50% of these are eventually published! Common reasons for rejection are listed in Box 11.1; compare your paper to this checklist *prior* to submission to try to avoid falling into these categories.

> ## Box 11.1 Common reasons for rejecting a manuscript
>
> - Poor introduction into research question with unclear relevance
> - Failure to review literature thoroughly at outset
> - Poor design
> - Small sample
> - Short follow up
> - Inappropriate statistics
> - Unjustified conclusions or overinterpretation
> - Poor synthesis of existing literature
> - Not conforming to target journal style
> - Poor targeting to journal
> - Sloppy work or writing

Reviewers are not infallible. It does not help to get angry by odd or contradictory reviews. You should look carefully at what has been written. Is it an outright rejection, or are they simply asking for clarification or suggesting an addition or change? Ideally, reviewers should indicate the importance of their points: which are essential and which are just suggestions? The editor may highlight a particular area or attempt to reconcile differing or contradictory reviews; addressing their comments is particularly important.

If you are invited to submit a revision, you are not obliged to make all changes suggested by the reviewers but each must be addressed in your response letter. If you disagree with a criticism or suggestion, you must clearly explain why. Ignoring a point gives the impression that something is being hidden. If you disagree with an editor's decision to reject a paper, it is reasonable to contest the point if you feel it is not justified but on no account try to push your luck or be aggressive. Most will be equitable if you have a case to make. If the reasons for rejection are sound, you are better off revising the work and submitting it to another journal than contesting the issue: you will waste far less time and the manuscript may be published sooner.

Presentations and posters

It is impossible to cover all the aspects of putting together a presentation or a poster within this chapter as they are large topics in themselves. It is likely that you will already have experience of doing presentations and even posters. However, there are a number of aspects related to preparation and delivery that should be touched upon. Furthermore, as seen in Chapter 6, there are points given on academic application forms for both types of presentation, and they are likely to be raised in interviews. In most circumstances, you will be presenting research that you aim to publish in some form in the future, so the process of presenting or making a poster is a very useful process in its own right.

Presentations

Being selected to present your research is a great privilege and is a perfect platform to project your findings to the wider research community either at a conference or meeting. Often you will have submitted an abstract to present at such an event so will have collected your ideas well in advance of receiving confirmation that your submission has been successful.

When preparing your presentation you must consider a number of factors:

* **Location and slides** – Whether your presentation is to a local, national or international audience, you will almost always be presenting in English as this is the universal language within the scientific community. However, particularly for presentations in non-English-speaking countries, ensure that you avoid using colloquialisms, and UK-specific abbreviations within your slides. Furthermore, be wary of using complex or advanced slide animations that may not be available elsewhere – if you are unsure, check before it is too late! The excessive use of animations can also be distracting, as can excessively 'busy' slides. Get your slides reviewed independently before the big day. This will not only help to ensure typographical errors are not

overlooked, but also that the slides are 'aesthetically appealing'. Take a back-up with you (on data stick or CD/DVD) or have it available somewhere on-line.

★ **Time** – Most presentations are time restricted to no more than 20–30 minutes. Some may be 7 or 12 minutes only. This is often monitored very closely and adhered to at meetings and conferences, so it is crucial that you bear this in mind. A suggested 'rule of thumb' for presentations is that you should not have more than one slide per minute of your allocated time. Having many more slides but talking faster is not a solution! There would be nothing more embarrassing for your presentation to be cut short in front of a room full of the world's leading experts in that area!

★ **Audience** – If you are presenting at a scientific meeting, you will have a mixture of academic, clinical and allied professionals present. You must be conscious of the level at which you are pitching. This is a fairly simple concept to deal with if you are presenting to an international audience on highly scientific subject matter, but less easy in other circumstances. The last thing anyone wants during a presentation is to send your audience to sleep! Avoid local colloquialisms and jargon.

★ **Questions** – The part of the presentation that everyone dreads! However, if you prepare well in advance you should be able to handle most questions. Remember you are the expert on your research. It is however useful to do a number of 'test runs' to uninitiated and unbiased audiences. Be conscious of the fact that often in conferences and meetings there may not be a general consensus or agreement on the theories you suggest from your research, so questions may be designed to spark further debate.

★ **Take home message** – This is the most important part of the presentation as this is what you want people to remember about your talk. Organise exactly what this message is, so it does not get lost during the course of the presentation.

Posters

The contribution of posters to increasing the communication of research between clinical academics should not be overlooked. Essentially it is a visual presentation of your research, which you can represent directly, and at the same time have one-to-one discussions with other interested researchers who come to read the poster. In many ways it provides a more intimate delivery of your findings in a less pressurised environment and at many conferences, your abstract will be printed within the conference abstract book too. There are a number of practical considerations when constructing your poster:

★ **Space available** – This varies from conference to conference so check the dimensions that are needed for your poster for this specific conference. It would be a disaster to turn up with a landscape poster when a vertical one was expected!

* **Layout of the poster** – The most aesthetically pleasing (and informative) posters tend to be those with less text, and more figures and tables. They are easier on the eye, can be read without needing to change your glasses prescription, and over the heads of a crowd of excited colleagues.
* **Font and spacing** – A 'busy' poster is very difficult to read, especially if the font is very small. Ensure it is well spaced out, and the font size is appropriate. Don't be tempted to overcrowd it – although it is a cliché, 'less is more'. Bullet points and succinct statements project the message you want better than continuous prose.
* **Title** – This will encourage interested parties to come and discuss your subject with you, so choose this carefully.
* **Take home message** – Keep it succinct, and directly to the point, so that those reading the poster know exactly what your findings demonstrate.

Beware!

* Don't leave printing your poster until the last moment – printers often need a few working days' notice
* Remember very bright colours may not project well on a poster, so check well in advance before it is too late

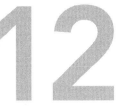

Research abroad

Stephen B Walsh
Cordelia EM Coltart

Many clinicians want to do research during their training for two major reasons: firstly, and probably most commonly, to improve their CV with papers and a higher degree in order to boost their job prospects, and secondly to dip their toe into the murky waters of academia, to see if academic medicine is for them. Doing research overseas can be an attractive way of achieving both of these aims and more, and one that the majority of trainees overlook when planning time in research. Indeed, those who have successfully performed their research abroad would argue that what's important isn't *what* you do your research on, it's *where you do it*! The world of research is constantly expanding and the possibilities for working abroad are endless. With a little determination and imagination during the organisational stage, working abroad is a hugely fulfilling and unique experience that can be both a life- and career-changing decision. This chapter will touch on a few of the more commonly trod pathways for UK doctors studying abroad.

Why do research abroad?

The appeal of working abroad is obvious from a lifestyle perspective – not only are you diverting away from your training programme for 3 years to pursue academic activities (which may be good for your physical and mental health), but the addition of doing it abroad has the potential to be a hugely positive life experience. It is a chance to improve your language skills, expand your cultural horizons, and even open doors to the possibility of building a career overseas. It may also be a chance to increase clinical experience in an area of research experience (e.g. HIV medicine in sub-Saharan Africa) thus broadening knowledge and developing your career.

Furthermore, just doing your research abroad is an unusual and impressive step and will immediately make your CV stand out from the crowd. Moreover, if you do your research in a non-English-speaking country, then it will be all the more impressive. Indeed, should you decide to try and make a career in academic medicine, then having strong links to a foreign centre is often very useful both for direct collaboration and for setting up links between hospitals and universities.

The major questions you need to consider are:

* Are the opportunities abroad greater than at home (e.g. excellent teaching, working with people you may have met before, areas with expertise in your speciality)?
* Will the extra time and effort required to organise a project abroad be worth it (e.g. where do you see yourself in 10 years' time and will it help your career)?
* Are there specific features abroad (e.g. research in the developing world, working in a world-renowned laboratory, prestigious institutions) that can't be obtained at home?
* Are there practical and logistical barriers to research abroad (e.g. financial implications of tuition fees, living costs, areas that are considered dangerous to foreigners)?

Possible research opportunities abroad

The scientific community is remarkably open, and research institutions are usually very happy to consider junior 'foreign' researchers joining them. This is not a selfless act as effectively applicants are an extra pair of (free) hands, who can usually be expected to write a number of publications in the 2–3 years of their time in that institution. In return, applicants should receive some research training.

The main opportunities can be broadly divided into three major areas:

1 **Developed world research** – Such as working in a world-renowned laboratory or working in a particular institution.
2 **Developing world research** – Such as working in rural institutions, where laboratory facilities may be limited but with increased access to major public health problems, infectious diseases etc.
3 **Speciality-specific research** – Working in specific environments that are unique to one specific part of the world, e.g. expedition research within the Arctic circle; space medicine research at NASA; working in areas where certain diseases are known to be specific to that region.

These opportunities may have a number of additional advantages. For clinical trials and for research involving human tissue, ethical considerations can prove extremely complex within the UK, whereas these hurdles are negotiated more easily in some centres around the world. Some UK universities have direct links with centres overseas or even help manage them, which can make life easier organisationally, e.g. Oxford University links with tropical medicine research in Vietnam, Thailand and the MRC centres in Gambia and Kenya.

Studying abroad

If you decide to study overseas, the type and level of degree (e.g. master's) need to be addressed in order to maximise the benefit to your long-term ambition. Take time to shop around and look at different courses. A good way to get further information is to contact the registrar's office or the office of student affairs, both of which are often happy to put you in touch with a current student or alumni to get further information. Be realistic about the likelihood of being accepted onto a programme and ensure you meet all the prerequisites. For example, graduate degree programmes in the USA require graduate entry exams.

As a trainee looking to do research, the model that holds in most countries is similar to the UK, namely that you'll enter the laboratory/research centre in a pre-doctoral ('pre-doc') position. You will also take up a project that will serve not only, hopefully, to generate publications but also give you training in research techniques and ready you to write up your work at the end of 2 years (for an MD) or 3 years (for a PhD). However, there are a number of countries around the world (e.g. China) in which a higher degree is increasingly seen as unnecessary, even for career scientists. Furthermore registering a PhD in an overseas university can be administratively difficult and expensive. Therefore, if planning research abroad you may be best registering this higher degree with a UK university and getting your PhD accredited in the UK. You will then have the benefits of a UK degree but the extra dimension of doing the hard work abroad. This is, of course, providing the research team you are working with are happy with that arrangement – it may be that centres elsewhere are measured by the number of 'pre-docs' they help advance through their PhD for example.

Beware!

By registering your higher degree in the UK you will receive accreditation from that institution if you are successful. However, remember this means you need to be in regular contact with that institution – including regular scheduled visits – which could mean expensive airfares!

What work to do

The first step is choosing the type of work you wish to undertake abroad. This may vary from clinical work to complement your academic training (in either urban or rural, developed or developing settings), to research (from pure scientific laboratory research to field-based population research) to studying for a higher degree. Other opportunities to work abroad in medically related fields include non-governmental organisations (NGOs), charities, governmental or medical relief work, although research possibilities may not exist in all these settings.

The most important factor is to be interested and enthusiastic in the work you are undertaking. Take time early on to think about what you want to get out of your time abroad; what is your primary objective? This may well determine which avenues of international work you wish to consider, e.g. if you are looking to come back to the clinical academic ladder in the UK with a basic science/translational scientific interest in a mainstream discipline, it might be wise to consider making links with centres of excellence in the developed world. However, if you are interested in pursuing your own esoteric speciality, global public health or international development, then 'field work' may be a more appropriate pathway. This may take the form of research in developing institutions, or medical officer/research roles for international organisations, NGOs or charities. Some of this will be pure clinical work overseas and some might be academic research, and it is important for you to know which you wish to do.

Where to do it

Developed countries

* **English-speaking countries** – Canada, Australia, New Zealand and the USA. The obvious advantage is that you can speak the same language, which will make any communication with potential supervisors easier. Experience will be similar to the UK in that most will have good facilities and universities. There may be an additional advantage of being able to supplement your income by practising clinical medicine in these countries. Culturally they are all pretty familiar and so, perhaps offer less in the way of expanding your horizon than work in non-English-speaking countries.
* **European non-English-speaking countries**, e.g. France, Germany, Spain, Scandinavia. These are rich industrialised nations, handily close to the UK. The university and research systems in these countries are broadly similar. Practicing medicine will be more difficult unless you're *very* good at speaking the language before you go. Regardless of your linguistic ability before you go, you'll come back fluent in the language!
* **Other highly industrialised countries** include Japan, Malaysia, Singapore and Taiwan. These countries have good facilities and interesting clinical material. Although in some areas language may be a problem, performing research here would certainly broaden your horizons. English is not necessarily spoken widely and travel back to the UK will also be expensive!

> **Useful information**
> Although research in China is rapidly developing, if you are considering research here a grasp of Mandarin or Cantonese is essential as English is not widely spoken, even in the science communities.

Developing countries

Important issues to consider when thinking about research in developing countries (e.g. Africa and parts of central and South America):

* With a few exceptions, laboratory facilities are likely to be poorer but opportunities for clinical research much greater. Money will probably be less of an issue due to the lower cost of living. For those interested in public health, tropical disease/infectious diseases, these countries contain a rich mix of clinical research material.
* Research in developing countries is less likely to be laboratory based and more likely to be epidemiological. You should also bear in mind that research in these settings might be difficult due to a lack of resources and infrastructure. It is therefore advisable to choose a location where some research facilities do already exist. For example, some funding agencies (e.g. the Medical Research Council (MRC) and Wellcome Trust or Oxford University linked centres) and institutions (e.g. London School of Hygiene and Tropical Medicine and Liverpool School of Tropical Medicine) have strong research collaborations with local institutions in these areas.
* Remote areas provide challenges of their own, especially social and scientific isolation. You will almost certainly need a supervisor who will support you from far away. This is in addition to regular visits to your UK institution to stay on track. It is also advisable to plan to do the write up in the UK, as you will need good facilities to achieve this (e.g. fast internet connections, libraries and frequent discussions with your peers).
* Speciality-specific research – This is a very niche area, with research usually being extremely difficult to plan but amazing if you achieve it!

▪ Is it even feasible?

Before making your mind up that research abroad is for you, you need to question whether it is even feasible in the first place. Box 12.1 summarises the main issues in more detail.

Box 12.1 Feasibility considerations to research abroad

1 Safety issues – Visit the Foreign and Commonwealth Office website for up-to-date information.
2 Immigration requirements – Visa requirements – Is a work permit required, cost of immigration process and timeline for these application procedures.
3 Professional requirement, e.g. level of language, registration of professional qualifications, are professional exams needed, cost of registration.

4 Impact of future career in the UK – Discuss this with your educational supervisor and training programme director.

5 Approval from deanery, training programme, GMC/JRCPTB/other Royal Colleges (applicable if you are planning on returning to the UK after placement).

6 Cost:
   - Travel costs – Airfare versus land transport if appropriate; number of journeys needed
   - Charges for tuition/attachment
   - Local living costs – Accommodation, transport, security measures, living costs (heating, lighting, electricity), telephone, internet, socialising, travelling, vehicle (if needed, plus petrol and insurance)
   - Funding options – Are there potential scholarships, grants, studentships, exchange programmes or can you afford to self-fund the venture?

7 Availability of living accommodation, secure location to live, e.g. whether accommodation is provided by the institution, proximity of location to facilities (shops, work and social activities). Note: In some circumstances secure accommodation may be needed where safety is an issue.

8 Income or wages – to supplement your funds, e.g. locum work, moonlighting, research assistantships etc.

9 Consider the impact on your personal circumstances and how well you would adapt to new surroundings.

10 Impact on your family, partner, children.

If you have a definite idea about what you want to do (and it is actually feasible), you need to make contact with the research group/principal investigators. If you have clinical academic supervisors who already collaborate with these individuals then this is a very useful way to make 'first contact.' Otherwise, you can usually contact most researchers directly yourself – email addresses are easily available from papers or university websites.

▦ Funding issues

Funding issues are discussed in greater detail in Chapter 9. However there are specific details related to research abroad that need to be considered. Indeed, this could well be the limiting factor in arranging a placement abroad. Often the posts are unpaid or have a significantly reduced salary, despite ongoing overhead costs for you and possibly significant relocation expenses. Therefore, you must calculate the anticipated costs carefully and budget accordingly. Unfortunately unless you are very lucky, funding is often crucial to being able to perform your research abroad. Of course, as in the UK, it is without question that a foreign research unit will welcome you with open arms if you already have your own funding in place – even more so if you have a full budget for a project. However, for the majority of people who do not already have a fully funded fellowship, funding for overseas research may still be better than staying at home.

Various countries have state-funded research programmes, notably the National Institutes of Health (NIH) in the USA. The NIH has an enormous budget and pays for international Fellows to come from abroad to work in US labs. Despite the recent global economic financial downturn, the NIH budget has increased!

In addition, doing research overseas can also open up specific grant money earmarked for international development or cooperation. There are many overseas development grants and fellowships offered by the Wellcome Trust and other such trusts. Scholarships and grants also exist for study abroad (e.g. Fulbright, Kennedy, Frank Knox, and BUNAC); although some are associated with restrictions, e.g. age limits. Likewise there are grants awarded by international bodies to foster cooperation; the British Council in France offers grants for young researchers working in France, for example. It is important to remember that many funding opportunities require application over 1 year in advance of the academic year you propose to begin studies. The UK Council for International Student Affairs (www.ukcisa.org.uk) and the Institute of International Education (www.iie.org) have comprehensive information on their websites. In addition you should contact your prospective universities/ research centres regarding funding opportunities for international students.

❗ Beware!

Funding opportunities abroad often require applications to be completed at least 1 year before you can start your research – be organised, or you could easily miss out!

Your potential supervisor abroad may also have a good idea of the best avenues to pursue for funding.

Supplementing your income while abroad

Starting research is often associated with a fall in your income when compared to the typical pay doctors receive when working in clinical environments in the UK. If you are doing research overseas, undertaking additional clinical work to supplement your income (as you may be able to in the UK) will be much more difficult. If you are going to an English-speaking country then working part time as a doctor may be fairly straightforward, depending on the institution. The USA will require you to take the US Medical Licencing Examination (USMLE), which may not be too hard to pass but it is quite expensive and time consuming. It is even harder if the country is not English speaking unless you are truly fluent in the language and the administrative or regulatory hurdles may be harder.

You may be able to supplement your income in other ways such as returning home for locum posts in the UK or even through teaching posts; in the end though it is likely that you just have to settle for less income during your research time abroad.

Families

If you have a family and/or children, doing research abroad will be harder. Those lucky enough to be going abroad with a fellowship will probably have money for dependants figured into the budget. Even so, asking your partner to find a new job in a different country, and moving children to a new school are big decisions, and for many they will be too much. Without a fellowship to cushion the blow, moving a young family abroad will be even more challenging. On the other hand a period of 2–3 years overseas, especially if children are young, can be extremely valuable, enjoyable and fulfilling as a family.

Other hurdles

Deanery approval

If you are planning research abroad you will need to apply for an OOPR (see Chapter 2) through the deanery and your training programme director in the same way as for research in the UK. If you are already in an academic post there will be protected research time available to you and with your training director's approval this can be taken abroad. The *Gold Guide* (www.mmc.nhs.uk) is a good resource to use when starting the investigation into what options are available to you. In addition, you need to decide if you want the time to count towards your training and if so get prospective accreditation. Again, there is no set format and this often varies between specialties, but a great place to start is to get the approval of your educational supervisor and your training programme director. The placement abroad will need to be deemed of 'educational value' in which you will obtain some of the core competencies required of your curriculum and approved by the relevant Royal College.

Box 12.2 gives a summary of common document requirements for undertaking research abroad.

Box 12.2 Documents needed when applying to undertake research abroad

- Passport – check the expiry date!
- Visa, work permit, licensing if applicable
- Evidence of professional and educational qualifications (e.g. transcripts)
- Medical clearance/documentation
- Vaccination certificates
- Medical insurance (plus or minus repatriation if appropriate)
- Letter of acceptance from supervisor and institution
- Evidence of funding

Key points

When planning research abroad:
- Be persistent! Obviously life is easier the earlier you start planning. This is the key to success as inevitably there may be setbacks. Be prepared to be patient and write a lot of emails!
- Consider carefully:
  - **what** type of work
  - **where** and **who** with
  - **feasibility**
- Do not underestimate the amount of time and effort it takes to organise logistics (processing applications, approvals, visas, work permits, licensing documents etc.)
- Consider carefully if this a cost-effective opportunity for your career and personal development at this stage

13

Common academic pitfalls

Arun J Baksi

Academic work can be richly rewarding both professionally and personally as well as being enjoyable and a source of great satisfaction. Some however find the very thought of research terrifying, daunting or simply tedious. Most of you will have friends and colleagues who have undertaken periods of research and will have likely heard a mixture of positive and negative experiences of academic life. This chapter aims to highlight some of the potential pitfalls that can occur in academic life so that you might avoid them. Many of these will not make or break a period of research, but can critically determine your experience and enjoyment of it. Much of this is common sense. It is worth being aware that difficulties can originate before you even start your research that will impact on what happens not only when you start but throughout your work.

Whilst publications and research have traditionally been required only for consultant and registrar (ST3) appointment in many specialities, these will of course mark you out in competitive specialities at an earlier stage. Even at foundation level some research experience or publications will help you gain the more attractive foundation training posts.

Some of you reading this will be excited by the prospect of a period of academic study and what it has to offer both in terms of your intellectual and scientific development as well as to the wider scientific or medical world. Others of you may see it purely as a hurdle over which you must jump in order for your career progression not to be limited and to remain competitive with your peers. Those in the latter group are particularly at risk of falling foul of the potential pitfalls of academic life (Box 13.1). Whilst some of these pitfalls are out of your control, many can be anticipated and avoided, or at least their impact minimised by anticipation, preparation, action or thought on your part.

Box 13.1 Summary of common pitfalls

Before starting
- Plagiarism/unoriginality
- Inappropriate project/supervisor/institution selection
- Timing of research within career
- Underpowering of a study
- Funding: Struggling with grant applications/failing to secure funding
- Ethics

During
- Lack of focus
    - Lack of discipline
    - Too diverse a range of academic interests/projects
    - Non-academic distractions/excess work to supplement income
    - Distraction by the Internet
    - Disillusion: with project/results/environment/lifestyle
- Lack of appropriate ethical approval
- Lack of structure
- Difficult supervisor
- Poor record keeping
- Introducing errors into data
- Failure to adequately back up data/work
- Losing funding
- Experimental failure
- Plagiarism
- Failure to write up before finishing

◼ Before starting

It may seem strange to focus on the period prior to starting full-time research, but in many ways, it is the preparation prior to a period of research that is most critical. It is at this embryonic stage that many potential pitfalls can be avoided. Before even committing to a period of research, let alone beginning it, it is valuable to ask yourself several questions:

★ Why am I doing this?
★ Am I suited to academic life?
★ What would I like to study?
★ Am I interested in my project?
★ What about funding?

In particular, it is wise to examine your motivation for and aptitude to research, which can require a shift in mindset from clinical work. If your heart is not in your research for whatever reason – be that the project, your supervisor, or for many other reasons, then it is worth considering carefully whether it is the right option for you before you commit to it. It is at the low points when you face difficulties, frustrations or disasters in your research that your motivation will be tested, and if this is found wanting, you may have insufficient determination to get through these usually transient but somewhat universal challenges. Very few projects are entirely free of adversity.

Important decisions and choices

Having decided to undertake a period of academic study, there are several important choices to be made. The most important of these are selecting your project and your supervisor, although it can be debated which is the more crucial:

* **Project** – The key element in this decision is to select something that interests you. It may be valuable to match your project to your subspeciality interest, not least to increase your training time in speciality-specific skills although this is not essential. Thought should be given to how data or any necessary samples will be acquired and in general, the less dependent you are on other people for this, the better.
* **Supervisor** – Choose your supervisor carefully – this can make or break your research experience and productivity. Select a supervisor who is interested in you and supportive of you. Of course they must be interested in the area of your project (it is likely to be in their research group) and ideally have relevant expertise and experience as well as time. Furthermore it is helpful if they have some incentive to support your progress. Ideally your supervisor will have a proven track record of successful supervision with students who recommend them and achieved good output. There can be tradeoffs between such things as eminence and availability for guidance such that some of the pre-eminent professors may not be personally available much of the time, but this is offset with invitations to help with their review articles and their established publication strength. It is also helpful to have a mentor for your wider career strategy as well as to support your research. It is worth considering how many supervisors to have. Whilst most people just have one, some have more. Both options have advantages and disadvantages and these depend greatly on the dynamics of each situation. Supervisors may contribute different areas of expertise or have different availability. Whilst multiple supervisors can be beneficial, if they have different objectives this can be highly problematic and there is a risk of you being caught in the middle of professional, political or personal conflicts.
* **Institution** – There are numerous influences on selecting an institution. Reputation is one, but relevant expertise in the area of your project is probably more important.
* **Timing** – It is worth considering how your research fits into your wider career plan not just in terms of topic, but also in terms of timing and training. Is it complimentary? Does it contribute to your training? Will the timing allow

you enough clinical time after completion of your research to optimise your skills by your Certificate of Completion of Training (CCT) date?

★ **Which higher degree?** – This will be influenced by multiple factors such as how long you wish to spend in research, whether you are planning an academic career, trends within your speciality, and crucially funding, as well as the preferences of your supervisor and institution. It is usually a fairly obvious decision and is best discussed with your supervisor or mentor.

Lack of originality

A thorough literature search is essential prior to planning your research. It is important that what is proposed is not a simple repetition of work already performed and published. Getting halfway through a project and discovering it has been done before can be devastating.

Plagiarism

It goes without saying that this is taken extremely seriously by institutions and if discovered can be hugely damaging, not just to your personal career and reputation, but that of your research institution and supervisors. It can lead to all your research being scrutinised and severe disciplinary action taking place against you. It can have major consequences for your academic and entire professional future. There are now sophisticated methods to detect this, made easier by the universal requirement for electronic submission of manuscripts and doctoral theses. In some institutions, regulations are emerging regarding 'self-plagiarism' and the ways in which your own work can be reproduced by you! One must also bear in mind copyright agreements made when a manuscript is accepted for publication. Whilst copying someone's data is clearly unacceptable, it is entirely reasonable to replicate work done by others in attempts to reproduce the results found or examine them further providing the idea is not claimed as your own. Given that this is a rather obvious potential pitfall, in this chapter I have focused on things that can be more insidious but equally destructive.

Funding and ethics

The more you have in place prior to beginning full-time research, the better. Funding and ethical approval should ideally be secured before beginning the full-time period of research as this can otherwise lead to significant delay and reduce the time you have for achieving your research goals.

During your research

Despite preparation, there is often a hiatus before full-time research can begin and this can be quite unsettling when accustomed to the constant and structured nature of clinical life. This transition can be troublesome and has the potential to derail you at the start.

Adapting

Switching from clinical to academic life can be challenging, as there can be quite a contrast. For many, this will involve starting work in a new place and new environment. You will have to establish yourself and develop a rapport with a new group of people, many of whom may be from a purely scientific background. Basic social skills and common courtesies are fundamental to this transition, e.g. offering to make tea for new colleagues. The onus is on you to both prove yourself (academically and socially) and forge relationships with the people around you. Both will have a dramatic impact on the remainder of your research time and can make all the difference, as this impact can be either positive or negative depending on the impression you create.

Failure to establish oneself in the academic environment as well as a sense of lack of progress can lead to a feeling of disillusion, especially in the first year. It is valuable to talk to friends and colleagues who are at a similar stage or have been through the process so you can gauge whether your circumstances or experiences are any different to theirs.

Choosing a basic science project throws up challenges that are often unfamiliar and can seem far from basic. It may be that only a small percentage of your experiments actually work, despite you feeling confident with the protocol you are using. In reality, only a small percentage of experiments will work as that is the harsh nature of science; if this is the case, actually you are doing extremely well. Your clinical skills will be mostly useless, you will be significantly less knowledgeable about the science than those around you and you may be much older than pure scientists.

Lack of focus and distractions

There are many potential distractions that can result in a lack of focus and ultimately lack of productivity. Perhaps wrongly, 'publication, publication, publication', is the mantra of academic life and productivity is the key measure by which you will be judged. Therefore it is always worthwhile considering what the outcome of any piece of work will be, specifically, will it result in a paper? You will be judged by output not intention and even the best of intentions can be detrimental. There are no prizes for unfinished work. It can be easy to take on too many smaller or side projects, especially whilst starting with your main project. As difficult as it can seem, it is important to learn how to say 'no', and developing a new assertiveness. Ultimately, you need to gain a higher degree and some published peer-reviewed manuscripts. Abstracts are attractive and relatively straightforward but it is peer-reviewed manuscripts that count for you, your supervisor(s) and institution. Progress and productivity can be maintained by trying to achieve something specific each day and by having specific targets. Furthermore, discipline is at the heart of academic success. Very few people in any aspect of life got anywhere without hard work.

The Internet can be both a blessing and a curse. Whilst information is only a few clicks away, so are a host of distractions. Much time can be lost checking email. Having email delivered to your phone can be an efficient way to avoid losing time to frequently checking your inbox. Alternatively, have a fixed time when you check email or making Internet usage a reward for achieving particular goals can be helpful strategies. Furthermore, succumbing to Internet distractions can be minimised by disconnecting your Internet connection whenever it is not required for what you are working on.

Beware!

If you're easily distracted by the Internet use a number of techniques to limit this distraction so hours of research time are not lost.

For most, a period of research will generate a lower salary than clinical work. Preoccupation with supplementing your income can result in significant distraction from research productivity. It should be remembered that the primary purpose of this time is research.

The context of these distractions is stark. Other groups may be working on similar things to you. Being beaten to a result or worse a publication is a serious adverse outcome. Do not delay writing up your work for publication by being distracted!

Handling data and losing it!

Accurate data is the foundation on which your research relies. It is therefore essential to keep accurate, organised and safe records of all data. It can be all too easy to introduce errors. Data error, corruption or loss can be catastrophic to a project, or at best create delay or frustration. Robust data backup is essential. The use of date- and time-named backups can avoid overwriting of new files with old or vice versa. Extra care should be taken to avoid data handling errors, particularly when working with large datasets or multiple data copies. It is often worth seeking advice from colleagues who are more used to handling data, and keep backups on different computers or university servers rather than single laptop computers, which are easily stolen. Do not forget to protect patient confidentiality if appropriate. Keep patient-sensitive data secure. Use password-protected files, encrypted data sticks and central servers rather than stand-alone computers or laptops and ideally no data should be kept together with patient identifiable details at all. This is your responsibility; breaches are taken extremely seriously and can result in disciplinary measures or even legal action.

Poor record keeping can lead to a multitude of difficulties. Besides data, records of ethical approval and consent should be maintained in a safe, organised and accessible manner in accordance with *Good Clinical Practice* guidelines.

Key points

When handling data, remember a few useful rules:

1 Keep a robust spreadsheet of your data, anonymised where necessary
2 Keep a robust backup(s)
3 Avoid multiple versions
4 Ensure you keep time-dated copies of documents
5 Ensure patient-sensitive data is kept securely at all times

Data ownership can also be an issue, particularly where funding is obtained from industry. Where possible try to maintain ownership of your data, at least institutionally.

Many projects will require you to learn new techniques, or use new software and for most of us statistics is a rather grey area. It is invaluable to engage with predecessors where possible to get to grips with new techniques. Many institutions now also run numerous courses or workshops in statistics, referencing software and research skills. This is extremely valuable, as when performing analyses such as power calculations, you need to ensure these have been done correctly whilst planning your research so that appropriate numbers of subjects are recruited within the timeframe of your work.

The difficult supervisor

Your relationship with your supervisor is crucial and it is worth investing time and effort into it. By and large, having agreed to be your supervisor, he or she has a vested interest in your success. As mentioned previously, careful selection of a supervisor minimises the likelihood of problems. Additionally, supervisors are less likely to be problematic if you create a good impression from the start and prove your reliability and productivity. However, despite all your best efforts the student–supervisor dynamic can be difficult. Therefore, it is worth speaking to previous students of your supervisor for advice.

Communication – as with most aspects of life – is fundamental to a good student–supervisor relationship. If you are struggling, then it is worth attempting to raise issues with your supervisor. If they are unreceptive, then you will need to identify the most appropriate alternative contact. Whilst supervisors can be demanding with hopefully beneficial effects on your productivity, it is important to recognise when requests or behaviour is inappropriate.

Although working with multiple supervisors can be fruitful, the dynamic between multiple supervisors can sometimes become strained, especially where the goals and motivations for the study have been wildly different. This atmosphere of 'too many chiefs' – often with competing or even conflicting interests – can have a negative impact on the progress of your research, causing delays and multiple problems for you. It is important that the interpersonal relationships between your supervisors are good and they have a common understanding of the purpose and structure of your work.

The supervisor who leaves

It is unusual for supervisors to leave whilst actively supervising projects, but this can occur and is somewhat out of your control. They may get promoted into a different university, leave for industry, or emigrate! It may be worth asking supervisors whether they have any plans to move when selecting them. If they do leave, the earlier you know, the better, so you can (jointly) plan how best to minimise the impact of this. It may be that they can continue to supervise you from their new location; you might move too or might transfer to an alternative supervisor.

Lack of structure

A structured approach to your research maximises your productivity and also creates a reassuring impression to supervisors and external observers. It is beneficial to produce a timeline for the duration of your research early on. Regular communication with your supervisor(s) not only keeps them up to date with your progress, but also helps direct your project as it evolves, although this can generate large quantities of additional work. It may be necessary to constructively decline additional work that may distract from your main project. Whilst your project might change course significantly during its progress, it is always worth keeping your primary objectives at the forefront of your mind and regularly appraising how well you are meeting these.

Grant applications and funding

A very common pitfall is struggling with grant applications and funding issues. This has been covered already in Chapter 9, but it is worth briefly touching on a few solutions to this problem:

* Try to get a copy of one or more successful grant applications to give you an idea about structure, content and style as well as paying close attention to the guidelines of the specific funding body.
* Do not hesitate to seek help from supervisors or colleagues.
* If you are repeatedly failing to be awarded funding, whilst this may simply represent the limited funding available with respect to the number of applications, it is worth identifying any factors within your control that may have contributed to this.
* Ask one or more people to review your funding application before you submit it.

It is extremely rare to lose funding once it is awarded providing you continue to satisfy the requirements of your awarding body. Some people start research without funding for the entirety of their work. This should ideally be avoided, particularly as much of the first year can be dominated by attempting to secure ongoing funding.

■ How to manage your day

There are as many models of a day in research as personalities, but two contrasting examples are given here. Consider which you might fall into and then plan how to avoid the obvious pitfalls!

Diary of a snoozer

'You snooze, you lose' – a bad day:

7.00am	Alarm went off. Pressed snooze.
7.10am	Alarm went off again. Pressed snooze.
7.20am	Alarm went off again. Still sleepy. Turned alarm off.
9.10am	Woke up. Now late. Jumped in shower and headed for station planning explanation for late arrival. Anxious wondering as to whether supervisor will be around?
10.10am	Arrived late. Walk of shame into the communal research office.
10.15am	Began first episode of cyclical checking of multiple email accounts.
10.45am	Made myself first coffee of the day. Chatted for half an hour with a friend about various things. Am still waiting for ethical approval so can't get on with project.
11.15am	Checked email again in case any mail had arrived. None in any of the accounts. Ordered some stuff online.
12.30pm	Early lunch.
2.00pm	Met with supervisor. Didn't get to discuss progress … thankfully. Agreed to undertake some other projects while waiting for ethical approval.
2.30pm	Checked email again before tidying desk.
3.00pm	Helped a colleague move some equipment for their experiments.
3.30pm	Asked a colleague for help with some power calculations, but they said they were too busy.
4.30pm	Left early to do some locum work. Every intention of having a more productive day tomorrow.
8.00pm	Got home. Dilemma as to whether to go out for planned dinner knowing I wouldn't enjoy it as day had not been productive or whether to cancel to work on stuff I should have done in the day. Managed to do neither. Had TV dinner and ended up watching a film I have seen five times all the way to the end.
12.45am	Film finished late so was after midnight before I got to bed. Alarm set for 7.
	Slept badly worrying about research, demoralised by work environment. Two days' work to do in one tomorrow....

Diary of an early bird

'The early bird catches the worm' – a good day.

7.00am	Alarm went off. Jumped on bike to work buoyed by yesterday's productivity.
8.00am	Began work in empty, quiet communal office. By nine o'clock had made great strides before anyone else had arrived. Supervisor stuck his head round the door and said 'good morning', noted I was in and working, but didn't distract me as he could see I was in the middle of stuff.
10.00am	Made coffee for colleagues around me and had a brief chat with one of them. Enjoyed finding out more about their work and them.
10.10am	Quickly settled back into morning's tasks. Identified further subject's for recruitment then prepared for today's experiment.
11.00am	Performed study on one of the subjects I recruited last week.
1.00pm	Enjoyed lunch after acquiring some great data.
1.30pm	Got on with analysis of the morning's data.
3.30pm	Discussed some of the day's data with my supervisor.
4.00pm	Asked a colleague for help with some statistics. They thanked me for making coffee in the morning and were happy to help. Got stats sorted with their help – thank goodness.
5.00pm	Got an email on my phone with final revisions of an abstract I had prepared and circulated for comments. Made relevant changes and submitted the abstract.
6.00pm	Left feeling very satisfied with the week's work so far. Booked a couple of weekend locum shifts as well on top of things. Cycled home and then went for a swim at the gym. Felt great.
7.45pm	Cooked dinner.
8.15pm	Did a couple of hours on a grant application and ethics submission for next bit of my research.
10.15pm	Arranged to meet a couple of friends for cinema and dinner tomorrow evening.
10.45pm	Went to bed looking forward to tomorrow. Relaxed with my novel before a good night's sleep.

Days can fall anywhere on the spectrum between these two days and can have elements of both in them. The more time you spend at one end of the spectrum the more likely your next day will be similar – and that can be good or bad depending on which day you are in. There is a desirable middle ground where conscientious and disciplined productivity allows for a reasonable work–life balance and satisfaction, enjoyment and productivity in your research. The more you are on top of your research goals and timeline, the greater your flexibility and ability to do additional academic, clinical and social activities with enjoyment and without compromising your research work. If you can establish a good daily routine early on, you put yourself on a path to success. The apparent hiatus experienced by many in the first 6 months of research can pose a significant threat to achieving this. Will you be the snoozer or the early bird?

Summary

Although this chapter doesn't cover every single academic pitfall it hopefully provides some simple guidance as to how to avoid the common problem areas and make your academic time more enjoyable and productive. One key consolation is that you certainly will not be alone in facing the challenges of academic life. A key piece of advice is to talk regularly to friends and peers within your own institution and at different institutions so that you can share and discuss experiences and hopefully find solutions to them and also so as to maintain perspective. With a little extra planning, anticipation and effort, many of the common pitfalls can be avoided and your research experience and output can be transformed.

Key points

Do:
- Learn to say 'no' so not to take on too much
- Avoid distractions – disconnect Internet!
- Aim to achieve something each day
- Talk to colleagues regularly
- Liaise with supervisor(s) regularly
- Be in control of as much as you can
- Try and write up your work before returning to a clinical work setting

Don't:
- Do something you are not interested in
- Overcommit yourself or diversify excessively
- Give up – keep persevering – it will be worth it in the end
- Keep quiet if you are struggling
- Lose sight of your primary goal

The future and the exit points in academic medicine

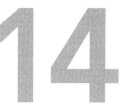

Opportunities in academic medicine after completion of clinical training

Gordon W Stewart

So you plan to embark on a career in academic medicine, meaning that you will be closely associated with, and probably employed by, a university rather than primarily the NHS. You may do this for one of two main reasons. Firstly, the 'research bug' may have bitten you, or secondly you may wish to teach in a medical school setting. Both of these activities can be combined and universities need both types of people.

◼ Determining your own future

By and large, the academic career is a very competitive one. There are a series of hurdles and each one has to be crossed successfully or you come to a halt. Furthermore, the crossing of the hurdle depends on satisfactory performance relative to the competition. In research your performance will be assessed by discoveries, publications and grants gained, of which the amount of money you can obtain in grants is the easiest to measure. In teaching, your performance is much less tangibly measurable but would include acclaimed excellence in delivery of teaching, student feedback and the successful organisation and delivery of a course, which might be part of the medical degree course, an MSc, or BSc or their modules.

Beware!

A sobering reality of an academic career is that you must get used to rejection quickly – applications for grants, fellowships and other senior positions may not always be successful first time around.

The great thing about an academic career is that it gives you an opportunity to be creative in one way or another. Within the NHS, you may be on a treadmill of clinics, ward rounds, management targets and asphyxiating bureaucracy. You are not your own boss and unfortunately you do not decide what you will do. However, in contrast, during the academic life you have greater freedom of action and are given much more scope to do your own thing. The best example of this freedom is when, on the research side, you run your own laboratory and you decide what experiments are going to be done and the future direction of your research. Similarly, on the teaching side you may be able to design a new course or even start a new medical school!

Apart from university employment other attractive routes for clinical academics may include:

* Working in the pharmaceutical industry.
* Working in public health or governmental/non-governmental organisations.
* Working in charitable organisations.
* Working in medical education/medical political organisations.

The world really is your 'oyster' but you do need a large slice of luck in addition to bags full of determination to reach your ultimate goals.

The long road ahead

Many people get their foot in the academic door at medical school. Outstanding academic achievements are very useful, but getting prizes at medical school is not easy. Some research projects at medical school can take off but you need not just a combination of hard work and effectiveness, but also a keen supervisor who is competent and has time to support you.

Currently a PhD is an almost essential requirement for an academic research career. However, if you are really good and were able to discover something important and publish it, then you could go forward without a formal PhD, although this is extremely rare. The typical route is to study for a PhD at some point after graduation, and in particular after you get a postgraduate exam such as an MRCP, although as discussed in this book already, there are many academic career routes some of which can start earlier than this. During your PhD you need to try to establish a core track record that says that you can do experiments, think scientifically and achieve results. Getting lots of publications out is great, but many feel the best kind of PhD is where you can look back and say, 'I discovered x, y or z'.

The postdoctoral period is exciting but no less challenging with competition for intermediate and senior fellowships being fierce, followed by the long path towards senior lecturer, reader and eventually professorial positions if you have been lucky enough to make it this far.

Roles and responsibilities

Senior lecturer posts

Typically you will have completed a series of jobs after the PhD (possibly fellowships/clinical lectureship posts), and be fully trained in a clinical speciality, be competent to work as a consultant of some kind, and be able to take responsibility for your own patients. To obtain successfully this type of post you will have needed to build on your PhD experience by performing further research projects and keep up your record of publication. Obtaining grants – and ideally a personal fellowship – will have provided a perfect opportunity and platform to perform more research in this type of position.

Easily the best senior lecturer position is a well-funded senior fellowship post, where your salary is often part-paid by a research funder, and where you have plenty of time for the research. If you can get one of these positions then universities will be desperate to accommodate you within their institution. Alternatively the more traditional senior lecturer position coupled with an honorary consultant contract (usually 50% time allocated to each function), is still a desirable option – but requires more balancing of clinical work with academic time.

When candidates are being reviewed for a senior lecturer post, the factors being assessed will include:

* The ability to obtain research funding in the future. This is the key condition. You will have to communicate that you have been involved in good science in the past, can see where you are going (and what is going on around you), as well as having a good track record that a grant funding body will be likely to appreciate.
* Depending on the job, the panel will also want you to be a safe (and preferably outstanding) clinician who will take some kind of interest in teaching students, although in a research-based job this will not be near the top of the list of essential requirements. Having at least done some teaching in the past will usually be enough, but during the interview, candidates will need earnestly and convincingly to say how much they enjoy teaching.

Reader posts

The title of a 'reader' is above the position of senior lecturer in the academic ranking system, although the responsibilities and roles are very similar. Essentially, a reader can be thought of as a professor without a 'chair' position – and requires evidence of an outstanding record of original research, as well as an excellent record of teaching and service to a university.

Useful information

Whilst working as a senior lecturer or reader, you may take on the following roles and responsibilities:

- Managing your own laboratory and clinical caseload
- Teaching or supervising other more junior academics
- In certain situations, you may concentrate entirely on research, doing no clinical or teaching work – you need to be good at grant writing to achieve this!
- Being involved in teaching but not to the detriment of grant writing and research, as it can be time consuming

Other local tasks include:

- Running graduate programmes, managing taught courses/degrees, running exams, organising the curriculum, mentoring of students, sitting on and chairing ethics committees
- Involvement in activities beyond your institution such as grant funding bodies, national or international groups with whom you share a research or clinical interest, and even into the Royal Colleges or the General Medical Council

---

Professorship – a chair

Seen by many as the pinnacle of an academic career pathway, a professor normally holds either a departmental chair (typically as head of a department) or a personal chair (awarded specifically to that individual). While most people who are promoted to professor simply continue with the activities that they were doing as a senior lecturer or reader, some take on senior management responsibilities, as chairs of departments or sections and in a few cases as heads of universities or medical schools.

Your role within academic institutions

It is extremely important for any organisation to have good people 'at the top'. A university chief needs to have vision and awareness of scientific, clinical, political and financial issues. Such a role also needs a decisive leader who will be brave enough to see through potentially unpopular but necessary paths, while always remaining diplomatic and fair to keep the many different groups of academics contented at the same time. Hence, in such senior positions, 'management skills' become essential, in addition to the academic and clinical skills that will have been developed over the preceding years on your career pathway.

As senior academics, your research and innovations will help to shape the success of the institution you work in as a whole. This has a positive feedback effect as success tends to breed success – attracting the best academics from across the world to want to collaborate or even invest financially or with expertise into your research. Therefore, senior academics must recognise how their research can benefit the wider institution and not just the individuals named on the publications.

Highs and lows

The clinical academic is unlikely to become very rich, although they are unlikely to starve too – substantial clinical excellence awards can bolster a successful academic's pay (additional payments made to consultants demonstrating hard work and excellence above and beyond contractual duties). However, only a couple of extremely talented academics will ever become as wealthy as an average surgeon in private practice. The summit of achievement in clinical academia is the contribution you make that influences clinical practice worldwide – and this only comes to a few. On a day-to-day basis the satisfaction of academia comes from the opportunity to have your own ideas and try and make something out of them.

Within the world of research it can be hugely demoralising to see your novel results published by somebody else before you get there. This can be very hard to reconcile with yourself and unfortunately it is part of the academic life. The other very common low is to have your grant application rejected despite a tremendous amount of work going into its submission. In contrast, it is hugely satisfying to have a grant application accepted and see your research ideas flourish with some exciting results. Either way, you must be able to cope with the low points and rejoice in your successes during your academic career to avoid falling off the roller coaster at any time.

Staying in the game

The key to a long career in academic medicine is being resilient enough to continuously overcome the hurdles and barriers on your route. On the research side you should try and keep up a steady record of publications. It does not really matter if the papers are in less well-known journals, but you must keep publishing! This helps to preserve your credibility. You just have to trust that one day, the really big publication will come. You also need to keep winning grant funding!

It is a very fine balance that must be achieved in academic medicine – juggling so many different responsibilities and roles. The ability to prioritise, delegate and cope with stress – as well as being able to say 'no' is crucial to maintaining your sanity. If you want to have a long and successful career, you cannot stretch yourself too thin as otherwise you will eventually break. The clinical academics that are best able to balance all the different facets of their career are often the most successful and the happiest in their jobs.

Key points

To optimise the opportunities in your academic career:

- Remember to keep focussed and decide which direction you want to head
- Remember this is a long career – ensure you do not 'burn out' too soon
- Accept that there will be highs and lows in this career pathway – the ability to cope with rejection is crucial
- Understand the roles and responsibilities placed upon career academics – both to their own research and to the wider institutions
- Do not stretch yourself too thin – you will break eventually!

15

Leaving academic medicine

David S Game

Leaving academic medicine might be an easy decision for many, but for most it is more than likely going to involve much soul searching. You may feel you are letting down your colleagues, abandoning your ambition or even upsetting your mum by markedly reducing the chances that she will have professorial offspring! You have to be true to yourself and the opportunities that arise, and this should not be a negative experience. Furthermore, you never really leave anyway.

■ Why leave?

This is often a difficult personal decision based on your own circumstances: let's assume you haven't been kicked out! There is rarely ever one reason, but the common ones are explored as follows. The reasons for leaving can be thought of as either internal or external.

Internal reasons

1 **Perception of job security** – This is probably the biggest reason for many, with money being a key determinant. Becoming a clinical academic already suggests that becoming rich is not a big motivator in your life. However, money is more important to some people than others. If you don't worry about money (or already have plenty) then job security might not be a big issue. The time to make the decision about whether to make the large step forward in academic medicine (for example to become a clinical lecturer/ senior lecturer) often coincides with starting a family and this can really focus the mind on income. As a woman especially in academic medicine, your focus at this time may also be on whether you can manage the work–life balance. Balancing a marriage, children, as well as stressful grant

applications every few years can be a fine art to master, but can induce understandable emotions of 'we can't spend the rest of our lives suffering every few years!'

2 **'Losing my religion'** – It can be exciting to experience the opportunities offered by a clinical academic job such as the clinical lectureship – you have a lot more exposure to the 'tripartite agenda' of clinical work, research and teaching. However, the challenges of working on your own academic programme can become increasingly time consuming and frustrating. At this time you have to question whether your ambition to succeed in this area is sufficiently strong to outweigh your perception of the challenges.

3 **Work–life balance** – Many people cite the pressure of clinical work, research and teaching as a reason to leave academic medicine. As mentioned earlier, if you add to this the time consumed with small children then this can be a major impetus to leave.

External reasons

1 **Research funding** – Applying for and securing research funding is essential for progression in the academic world. However, in this current financial climate the possibilities for future research funding are looking bleak, with some research councils writing off huge areas of previously funded research. Even without this added economic pressure, being an academic will require you constantly to apply for new grants, support your research group and generate income.

2 **Behaviour of Higher Education Institutions (HEIs)** – Over the last few years the response of most HEIs to the adverse economic climate has been a difficult process. Implementation of cost-saving restructuring of academic departments has led to some extremely difficult working conditions and a number of job losses. Even very highly respected academics have come under pressure: tenure is unfortunately dead. While it is accepted that there is a need for performance management, many academics have expressed concern over the mechanisms by which some HEIs manage these changes, especially for clinical academics who are always split between clinical and research obligations.

3 **Opportunity elsewhere** – Consultant positions are hard to come by, especially in the most sought-after posts. Despite the many years of struggle and toil within a hospital speciality, when and where you get your consultant job can largely depend on luck and good timing. Therefore if you are thinking of leaving, and an opportunity arises, it can sometimes be 'too good to refuse.'

Beware!

Despite having an excellent track record in clinical academic medicine, application to higher fellowship/lectureship positions is not guaranteed – the competitive process continues!

■ How to leave

The easy way to leave (i.e. not turning up to work) is definitely not the best way! You may want to consider the following options:

1 **Carefully consider ongoing grant applications** – This will depend on what you have submitted and how certain you are about leaving. The obvious advice is to weigh up how much work is required to submit grant applications against your likelihood of leaving. If you are still undecided and you can update a previous grant proposal then you should probably go full steam ahead and get the application in. Depending on the sort of grant you apply for, there may be an opportunity to take some of the research funding with you even if you leave your current post. Conversely, if you are pretty sure that you aren't staying then there may be much better ways to spend your time than writing a grant proposal from scratch.

2 **Assess your CV** – If you are in any doubt about continuing in academic medicine, you must make absolutely certain that should you decide to leave, you have the best possible chance of securing another job. If you are leaving with significant time left in higher training then you should be easily returned to the clinical training scheme, but you still need to look forward. Fortunately, most medical academics look good on a consultant job application form: you will have a higher degree, publications, international presentations, teaching experience and other transferable skills. In fact in some ways it is rather unfair on your non-academic colleagues with whom you are in competition that you are applying for the same job. However, given the lack of a level playing field, you should ensure that it is as un-level as possible! You must write up your thesis in good time for the job application. You need to be ruthlessly efficient in making sure you have written up all publishable research and have at least presented abstracts in any work that is unlikely to be fit for publication by the time you finish. You should already have attained a teaching qualification, but if not should try to make the most of any opportunity to do so. Even if you fail to complete this in time for the consultant interview, it will give a positive impression of your commitment to this area.

3 **Finding the job** – You will probably have been keeping your ear to the ground for some time and have an idea about what is going to be coming up. If not, then you have some work to do: use all known contacts to learn where and when jobs will be coming. If anything sounds good, make an appointment with the clinical director or clinical lead; be enthusiastic and ask to be kept updated with any progress and timing of job advertisements. Beware of promises about jobs though – many have thought the job had their name on it and been disappointed later.

4 **Speak to your boss** – You should have an academic mentor who is independent of your immediate boss – this is your first port of call and you should be able to have an honest and confidential conversation with them. In terms of your

real boss, the timing of discussions about leaving will depend upon how sure you are that you want to leave. If you are absolutely certain then you should probably speak honestly as soon as possible; if you are not sure then you might want to wait. This decision will also depend on the sort of relationship you have with them: a detached senior academic might not be very impressed with wavering ambition but if you know them well then there shouldn't be a problem.

5 **Applying for the job** – This is really the realm of an interview course and cannot be covered in great detail in this chapter. However, as with academic applications, make sure your application exactly matches the job description. If you have a very academic CV and the application is for a pure 'service provision' NHS consultant post, then make sure your application form and/ or CV is written accordingly – it will look quite different to the CV on your grant applications! Furthermore, make sure you do your homework and find out as much as you can about the organisation in which you hope to work. Finally, make the most of the pre-interview visit – you may find that this is your real test, not the interview.

6 **Inform your HEI and/or funding council that you are leaving** – Only do this once you have a job!

Key points

Do:

- Speak to your mentor as soon as possible
- Be realistic in finishing research projects
- Make your CV stand out from the rest
- Actively look for job opportunities

Do not:

- Just stop doing experiments/research
- Withdraw from teaching responsibilities
- Be miserable or resentful

Life after academic medicine

The chances are that you will have been selected for your new non-academic job on your strengths rather than weaknesses. This being the case there may well be an expectation on you to perform in teaching and possibly even research to a limited degree, and probably in that order to begin with. This is the perfect scenario: you can incorporate the work you love outside of direct clinical care into a job plan. In theory this means you actually get paid for what you do, which seems a bit alien to the expectation of ever-increasing teaching workloads as a medical academic, when your research may suffer as a consequence. If you work in an academic health sciences centre, then the roles and responsibilities of NHS versus university employees are increasingly blurred: in some ways you can have your cake and eat it. Clearly this will be different in primary care as a self-employed general practitioner or as a district general hospital (DGH) consultant.

W hether you are returning to a training rotation or to an NHS consultant post, your professional life will be permanently transformed by your experience of academic medicine – in many ways you never really leave.

Further reading

Justice AC. Leaky pipes, Faustian dilemmas, and a room of one's own: Can we build a more flexible pipeline to academic success? *Ann Int Med* 2009;151(11):818

Lederman D. (2007) *Why women leave academic medicine.* Inside Higher Education. Available at: http://www.insidehighered.com/news/2007/09/21/women

Lowenstein SR, Fernandez G, Crane LA. Medical school faculty discontent: prevalence and predictors of intent to leave academic careers. *BMC Medical Education* 2007;7:37

Index

Abbreviations

ACF   – academic clinical fellowship
CL   – clinical lectureship
OOP – out-of-programme
OOPE – out-of-programme for experience
OOPR – out-of-programme for research